Mobilizing Your Healing Power

Mobilizing Your Healing Power

Discover Abundant Healing Energy

James L. Kwako, M.D.

ISBN 0692794247
ISBN 13: 9780692794241

The cover: Just as the sunrise shines on us all, so, too, is the power of the light, love and joy available to all with eyes to see. The task is to take the light and energy of the higher self into the shadow areas to heal them into wholeness.

Dedication

This book is dedicated to the divine design of healthy well being in each of us.

Acknowledgements

I wish to thank all those folks who put their trust in me to be their physician. I appreciate the many stories that have been shared, some of which are included in these pages.

I appreciate the mentors who have shaped my career. At the beginning was Bill and Gladys McGarey, the husband-wife team that courageously confronted conventional medicine. They hosted an annual meeting that was part of the frontier of holistic healing that explored and explained how to use many tools of healing. They studied and supported my research into the healing power of dreams, acupuncture, intuitive healing and reincarnation.

Norm Shealy, M.D., Ph.D. taught me how to grasp the power of holistic principles of healing, organize them in a coherent fashion and compel those who would listen to apply them in their lives. He taught me how to teach wellness, to project optimism and instill the will to heal. During my time with him he founded the American Holistic Medical Association that brought together a wide array of like-minded professionals on the cutting edge of medicine. His prodigious energy and intensity was infectious on a daily basis.

Evarts Loomis, M.D. founded Meadowlark, a residential retreat center that dedicated to whole person care. This experience with him enabled me to be part of a multidisciplinary group healing endeavor that effectively changed lives. I especially learned from his enthusiasm and eagerness to explore every avenue of healing and share it with as many as possible who would listen. It was a high honor to be part of this healing center model of the future.

During many of these years unfolded a relationship with Robert Leichtman, M.D. He is a highly intuitive physician, author and teacher of spiritual principles of living. I deeply appreciate his wise counsel in handling the challenges of a busy practice, teaching principles of healthy living and raising a family. His insight and inspiration explores may aspects of the spiritual path and how to integrate it into daily living.

I especially need to thank my sister Marilyn Ehreth and Jack Canfield. When I introduced Jack for a monthly integrative medicine study group he made the comment that there was a book in that statement. I essentially said that healing is a physical sense of wellbeing with energy, strength and vitality. Emotionally it is the presence of enthusiasm, compassion and cheerfulness. Mentally it is an active mind that is curious, eager to learn and determined to make a difference. Spiritually it is being dedicated to a larger purpose, to serve the soul and the groups to which we belong.

A few week later I had a dream in which I was walking with my sister, Marilyn. We walked up a hill and then suddenly I was carrying a baby on a frozen body of water. People were ice fishing. I thought how terrible it would be if the baby crawled into a fishing hole and fell into the ice cold water. Suddenly the baby was under water and about to die. I recovered the baby and walked toward a warm house.

Upon reflecting on the dream it soon became apparent the baby was the new idea of writing a book, that if I don't pursue it soon it will die like a baby under water in an ice cold lake in winter. Within a few days I began to write and a few years later put finishing touches on the many steps taken.

I appreciate the support of my wife, Jamie, and children, Alex and William, for their patience and tolerance of a busy medical practice, teaching and writing. They have been lovingly supportive over many years and have brought me the delights of countless family events, celebrations, major decisions and enjoyments which infuse many of these stories and ideas.

Table of Contents

Introduction

I have been an active physician for over 40 years. During this time I have seen a great deal of suffering and a wide range of disease. Trained as a conventional physician in Family Medicine, I see all ages, young and old, men and women, with acute and chronic disease, from mild to severe. Compared to only 100 years ago, modern medicine is filled with miracles, and I have seen many of them. Infections like pneumonia and appendicitis used to be major causes of death but now are healed daily. Heart attacks, serious arrhythmias and stroke are often treated successfully. Blindness and deafness are amazingly treated, at times reversed and often prevented. Many forms of cancer can be successfully treated and life extended far longer than before. A great deal of prevention of heart attacks and cancer occurs daily. Modern medicine is developing extraordinary ways to detect disease tendencies at birth with DNA and genomic studies. In the near future the main emphasis will be on prevention. We are living longer with greater quality of life than ever before.

I am grateful to be a physician and a member of the healing arts. I see healing occur every day, lives being saved and life being prolonged due to expanding science and the sacred art of healing. Most of all, I am fully aware of the potentials for how life can be made better, however short or long it may be in the body.

However, beyond the use of medications and surgery, medicine today, lacks guidelines for how to heal yourself. It is mainly authoritative and arrogant. It is just beginning to be collaborative which is the essence of healing. Each of us needs to learn how we became ill and how to access sources of healing, especially serious and chronic disease. Most of all we need to learn how to be well in body, heart, mind and spirit. We need to learn how to enjoy and rely on vibrant health for a full life span with minimal aches, disease and distress. We should be able to look forward to a future of growing health in our career, family and special interests, especially as we age.

Physicians are trained to look for physical symptoms and signs of problems not signs of stress and distress that often lead to and trigger disease. And far too many are not only skeptical but critical of those pursuing healing methods and wellness medicine beyond current standards of care. Too many are still stuck in a rut of narrow and close-minded medicine.

Unfortunately physicians are almost exclusively trained to address acute disease and life-threatening illness. While this is often the proper priority, there is much more to healing. Chronic disease is far more common as we age and dealing with it is the current greatest need for quality of life. Overweight affects over 60% of us, obesity in over 30%. Chronic pain is present in up to 55% of us. Fatigue is very common in those over 40 years of age. Conventional medicine is just beginning to address these even though millions are already suffering from them.

Fortunately, the healing field of medicine is expanding even further than conventional medicine. Integrative medicine is the new specialty bringing together alternative and traditional approaches into the mainstream. Integrative approaches study and prescribe healthy ways of living and how to best use nutrition, micronutrients and hormones for optimal health. Food testing is far more specific and beneficial than ever before. We study stool specimens that reveal the normal flora in ways that lead to successful treatment in many whom conventional medicine is unable to help. Hormone testing is far more comprehensive and effective than the usual testing and treatment allow. There are now many tests available to help identify risks for cancer and practical dietary suggestions that can help us prevent it.

Mobilizing Your Healing Power

Early in my career I had the wonderful fortune to meet and work with brilliant physicians on the cutting edge of medicine and the healing field. Soon after my medical training I had the unique opportunity to work at a chronic pain clinic founded by C. Norman Shealy, M.D., Ph.D. He is a neurosurgeon who has made major contributions to the field of chronic pain, stress management and wellness medicine, and the founding President of the American Holistic Medical Association. At this clinic we offered a thorough medical evaluation, frequent therapeutic massage, gentle spinal adjustment, acupuncture, extensive counseling and neurological reprogramming. We also incorporated remarkably effective medical intuitives and healers into the program to help with diagnosis and treatment. The most effective part of the program was the nerve retraining through relaxation, visualization and meditation exercises. The experience at the Pain and Health Rehabilitation Center opened my mind in many ways to empower healing with intense affirmation, creative imagination and invoking the will to heal. This was a remarkable experience to see people heal chronic disease, especially pain and stress disorders, reverse major medication use and regain a new lease on life.

Right after my residency in Family Medicine I had the extraordinary experience to work with Bill and Gladys McGarey. They were a husband-wife physician team that established the Edgar Cayce Medical Research Center in Phoenix, Arizona. They inaugurated the use of the brilliant healing perspectives of the Edgar Cayce work. Mr. Cayce was declared in the New England Journal of Medicine as the pioneer of holistic medicine in the 1970s. His incredible depths of insight foresaw organ transplants in the 1920s as well as the enormous value of intuitive assessment to diagnose complicated diseases accurately. He diagnosed many illnesses with a depth of perception that we are barely beginning to comprehend today.

The McGareys helped to apply Mr. Cayce's awareness of the subtle energy bodies that are the source of health and disease. As the bodies of matter, emotion and mind are uplifted we can invoke the real power of healing energies that does make a difference over time. With them I learned about basic principles of acupuncture, nutritional medicine, prayer and dream work. At times there were rapid cures. Most of the time we learned to be patient and content with finding and knowing a path toward healing. This in itself was deeply reassuring to most of those with a chronic ailment, fear or frustration.

I also had another extraordinary opportunity to work at Meadowlark Retreat Center. It was a residential whole person treatment center founded by Evarts Loomis, M.D., dedicated to medicine of the whole person. Guests came all over the country and often from other countries. They stayed one to four weeks at a time. One-third attended the center to address serious medical problems like heart disease, chronic pain and cancer. One-third came to confront emotional distress associated with marital problems, job stress, or grief from loss of a loved one. The rest came to renew themselves, lose weight or re-evaluate their direction in life. Several classes were available each day including yoga, movement to music, art expression, journal writing and meditation. There was also a fasting group that attended a morning awareness class which emphasized dream interpretation work.

Meadowlark was a fascinating experience that allowed the chance to see accelerated healing occur in many. It often took three to four days for guests to separate themselves from the usual daily routines and seriously begin to focus on themselves. Many stories of insight and personal revelation unfolded during this time, convincing me of the healing power potential within all of us. I was medical director there for about ten years.

Beyond conventional scientific medicine is a vast field of scientific wellness medicine that focuses on the principles of how to be healthy in body, heart, mind and spirit. Each of these parts of ourselves has an important role to play in our basic health and well-being. Each has an innate life requiring attention for full function and fruitful expression. And each has several systems that uniquely add energy, goodwill, alertness, intention and purpose. The body has organ systems for the brain, heart, hormones, lungs, intestines and more. The emotional body has negative psychic zones such as fear, doubt, anger, and resentment as well as positive zones of kindness, caring, courage and goodwill. The mind embodies the skills of organizing, remembering, relating and pondering the ideal as well as the potential for narrow-mindedness and blind beliefs. The spirit has immense reservoirs of purpose, power and perspective; its only limit is in not being used. These are all designed to work harmoniously together to most effectively integrate the higher energies with the lower ones to increase our effectiveness in living.

The goal of full health is to have each of these dimensions working as well as possible. The purpose of well-being is to express our unique perspective, participation, and loving presence to those with whom we live and work. The ultimate goal is that we fulfill our missions for living and do so with as healthy a body, heart and mind as possible. Most of us can do better. This book is my effort to show how we can.

After a brief discussion of causes of disease and principles of healing, I have divided this book into four main sections. For physical health there are chapters on nutrition, exercise, energy, the use of supplements, hormones, and sleep. For emotional maturing there are chapters on stress, relaxation, relationships, and resistance to healing. For mental agility there are chapters on memory medicine, enlightened approaches to work, exploring the meaning of dreams and increasing intuition. For the spiritual aspects of healing there are sections on communing with nature, prayer, meditation, death and the afterlife.

This book addresses the whole person body, mind and spirit. It draws upon the experiences of thousands of patients, scientific studies, professional observations and personal experiences. The uniqueness of this book is that it encompasses a holistic view to medicine and healing. Our body, heart, mind and spirit each have important roles to play in our overall well-being. Within each of us are layers of function from the concrete physical to gradually increasing subtle levels of beauty, love, wisdom and joy.

Mobilizing Your Healing Power is written to show how the finer aspects, expressions and attributes of life are integral parts of our everyday world and the energy of healing. We are each meant to grow into higher elements of our self-awareness and self-expression to make a healthy contribution to the lives of those around us. The book will help you learn how to take care of yourself, promote self-healing and add to the healing of others. It reveals the abundance of healing resources available to each of us and offers practical guidelines for how to activate them.

Chapter 1

Causes of Disease are Not Mysteries

The cause of an illness is always worth considering. Finding the cause does not ensure the cure but it is usually helpful. Many people with a cough or sore throat are glad to hear that it is a cold virus not a flu virus or strep throat or pneumonia. When suffering a pain problem there is always relief at knowing the cause is a muscle strain rather than deeper damage in the kidney, abdomen, lungs or heart. Knowing that the cause of disease is milder and familiar releases or prevents expressing energy on common fears, worries and deeper concerns.

Knowing the cause of serious problems is important because it provides a name, a focus and, hopefully, a body of knowledge and direction. We hope that finding the cause connects us to a source of understanding and healing. Unfortunately, serious conditions, even when diagnosed correctly don't usually have simple solutions. Invariably they require a multi-stepped approach to new learning, growth and healing. However, being on the path of healing is always better than a path of disease, distress and depression. Going toward healing is always more reassuring than deteriorating toward greater pain and depression. Small degrees of success are always worth celebrating.

Fortunately there are many common causes to most problems that are worth knowing, accepting and integrating into our daily health routine. The big picture of causes helps reassure us that we are not only treating disease and distress but also preventing unnecessary problems from occurring.

The Common Causes of Disease Are Infection, Strain, Aging, Genetics and Lifestyle

The most common infections are viral. The common cold hits many people averaging three times per year in the adult and five times per year in children. The flu virus is definitely more debilitating, though usually still mild with only about 10% each year succumbing to a more severe reaction. Severe disease can occur from viral infections that are now being implicated in triggering chronic fatigue, irritable bowel syndrome, thyroiditis and at least a few tumors. Bacterial infections respond well to antibiotics in most circumstances though resistance to them is a real challenge for serious and chronic infections. Fungal infections are common though mostly mild with only occasional exceptions.

Louis Pasteur is the pioneer of bacteriology, finding the bug as the problem. However, he also said that the condition of the organism is more important than the presence of the infecting agent. It is not the destructiveness of the bug that is as important as the health of the body it invades. This means that the state of the immune system and the body as a whole is a major determining factor in whether an infection invades and/or becomes serious. Our current state of health or lack thereof determines our risk for infection. The healthier we are the lower the risk we have for infection. Thus the key to causes of infection is often the health we do or do not have to begin with. Major questions to find the cause should include the state of health in diet, exercise, mood and mind before the problem arose.

Over-exertion strain, repetitive injury and physical accidents lead to much suffering and chronic pain. As my own body ages I am all the more aware of what I have been seeing for years in many others. Minor injuries are annoying and heal faster when we are younger. Major injuries occur more easily, can be debilitating and often do not heal completely as we age. Most of us do not appreciate the health we have until it is missing and therefore are not dedicated enough to keep it in good condition. In addition we are not careful enough to consider the strain we put it through, assuming that what the body used to do with ease at an earlier time can be resumed at a later time in spite of less strength, agility and stamina.

A simple stretching exercise routine is sufficient to treat 70% of back strain problems. This means that lack of exercise should be considered a primary cause of acute and chronic pain conditions. There are a wide variety of stretching routines. It almost doesn't matter which one is chosen as long as it is done once or twice a day. If exercise is so effective for reversing muscle aches and pains how much more beneficial would it be in preventing such conditions?

Aging occurs in all of us but can always be improved and sometimes reversed The peak of health in most of us is in the 20s unless you are in gymnastics when you perform best in the early teens. The average age in men has increased in the U.S. to 75 and to 80 for women. As a result of increasing longevity many other conditions have become apparent, especially heart disease and cancer. As the body ages all of the organ systems lose some efficiency, maintenance and regeneration capacity. Although some of us are far more prone to illness than others, the body is more fragile and does not repair as well as we age. Fortunately there are many ways to minimize the changes of aging, but it remains a major cause of much distress and disease.

For practical purposes of quality of life, the main changes of aging involve loss of energy due to nutrient and hormone deficiencies. We often do not adjust our nutrient needs with later phases or new circumstances of life. As a result we do not provide our body with the vital nutrients for most effective function and vitality. Our digestive and assimilative activities diminish requiring food and supplement changes to maintain them. If just the endocrine system is optimized many more would feel better longer and with less disease. Lack of hormone health increases our risk for disease and is one of the causes we unknowingly set in motion.

Our genetic background plays a role in causing disease. We are all affected by the genes of our parents and their families. It is always worthwhile reviewing family medical history to consider our own potential risk conditions. Gene studies are the current growing peak of medicine. We are identifying a wide range of illnesses related to specific genes and gene combination disruptions which are closely connected to optimal use of medications, supplements, hormone levels and a healthy lifestyle. Whether these develop or not depends on how well we take care of ourself and how we react to life's challenges. Less care results in a greater likelihood that disease promoting genes become more active and health-promoting genes less active.

An unhealthy lifestyle is the cause of most physical disease. Inadequate nutrition, exercise and stress management lead to many common conditions as well as serious ones. A growing number of studies estimate that diet has a the major role in decreasing heart disease and cancer, which is roughly 50% worse in those with poor diets. Studies also show their role in intestinal problems, chronic pain and various types of arthritis.

The obvious causes of poor nutrition in the West are the over-consumption of foods without optimal nutrient content. Fast foods are high in fat and calories without the essential proteins, fats and carbohydrates. There are healthy and unhealthy fats, carbohydrates and proteins. The challenge is to learn how to choose the best in each category. With the older population a growing concern is depletion of protein and many micronutrient vitamins and minerals due to low intake or deficient digestion.

Over the last hundred years a major cause of disease is a lack of adequate exercise extending from childhood to older age. Insufficient diet and exercise should be considered the two most relevant and reversible causes of lifestyle related disease.

An unhealthy lifestyle must also account for the inability of most of us to handle the stresses, worries and frustrations that we all experience. Stress itself has been widely quoted as responsible for about 70% of illnesses. This number is hard to verify. However the physical stress disruptions are medically well-known, affecting every organ of the body. A lack of how to respond to life's demands should be considered a major cause of disease. Our reaction to stress is usually more important than the stress event itself.

I also suggest that we consider a host of psychological malfunctions as lifestyle precursors to illness. These would include prominent levels of fear, self-doubt, chronic worry, grief, and anger. It is common to experience these in many ways as we go through life's challenges. They become part of the cause when sustained over lengthy periods of time without at least partial resolution and healing. Major psychic turmoil requires a concerted focus to heal otherwise we consume large amounts of energy and attention.

Needless to say, an unfulfilling career and/or relationships should be considered causes of distress and disease. Hating work or a close family member is like seeding cancer in the emotional body. It will amplify weak links of the body and lead to disease of some kind as well as accelerate the whole aging process.

A healthy lifestyle is the key to overcoming most causes of disease and loss of well-being. A healthy holistic lifestyle embraces physical, emotional, mental and spiritual practices for optimal health. The more we develop ourselves in a balanced way at each of these levels the more healing energy is mobilized to ensure health, vitality and successful living. Each of these is a vast field of energy and purpose.

The physical realm includes diet, exercise and how we use the body. The emotional self includes the wide range of feelings that are unpleasant and distressing to the more enjoyable and beneficent. The mental body includes many skills of mind from organizing and planning to intuiting and extracting the subtle meanings and joys of life. The higher self, the self's best self, is the source of our identity and wellspring of our divine design, the driving force that propels the best of who we are. As we expand the best within each of these major departments of ourselves, we draw forth healing energy and radiate it to those around us.

Physical Causes of Disease

The body enjoys being well. It knows the value of vitality and efficient functioning. It is like riding in a new car, all the parts are performing as designed. There is a smooth hum to the engine and each action of the car from starting to turning to accelerating and stopping. When all the organs are optimally functioning the many activities of the day are smooth without stiffness, tiredness, achiness or slowness. When the body is not well it breaks down in many ways. The causes for the loss of physical health are many, the simplest of which is the role of nutrition.

A poor diet can lead to disease of every organ of the body. The most common conditions due to a poor diet are intestinal such as heartburn (which is related to GERD, reflux esophagitis and gastritis), irritable bowel syndrome, constipation, bloating and indigestion. However, it is worth noting that a wide variety of other organ systems are also worsened by poor food ingestion and digestion such as heart and blood vessel dysfunction, headaches, fatigue and many skin problems.

The main problem most of us have in this country is overconsumption malnutrition. The foods that are most likely to cause problems are excess amounts of nicotine, sugar, salt, fat and alcohol. These quickly stimulate a pleasant taste that becomes a preference and then becomes a habit. However, they do not have the nutrient content complex of vitamins, minerals, essential fats, essential protein and optimal carbohydrates. We have sufficient calories with insufficient micronutrients that causes depletion of tissue building and regeneration actions. With minimal strain or stress the body cannot keep up with the maintenance needed. It more easily wears down, becoming vulnerable to infection and injury.

Insufficient exercise is a cause of most musculoskeletal pain problems. Lack of conditioning increases the risk of injury and minimizes repair capacity. One hundred years ago almost everyone was physically active enough. Today, most of us are not, and lack of conditioning contributes to most disease. It must be considered a cause of organ depletion, immune dysfunction and general lack of stamina.

Less mentioned but worth noting is that physical exercise increases our sensitivity to judging whether a certain activity is easy to do or a risk of overstrain. The better shape of our body the more likely we respect its ability to perform certain tasks and thereby work within our reasonable limits to do so.

The greatest cause of physical disease is emotional distress. The reason is because we do not know how to separate feelings of distress from body functions. But there is a difference between the body of matter and the body of feeling. If not constrained to the body of feeling, distressing fear, worry and anger will adversely flow into and affect the physical body. Stress increases nerve energy to the heart, brain and muscles, and decreases energy to the abdomen. As a result we are more prone to over-excitement of these organs resulting in physical problems. Over-strained muscles result in tightness, constriction and pain. An over-working heart increases the risk for hypertension, heart irregularities and maybe chest pain from coronary spasm. A super stimulated nervous system leads to anxiety, insomnia, headaches and cognitive dysfunctions such as impaired memory and concentration. Under stress there is less circulation to the abdomen leading to decreased digestion, assimilation and elimination.

Misery Mood Makers

Dysfunctional emotions lead to mood disorders in addition to physical disease. There are a wide variety of emotional disorders many of which can be separated into over reactions or excessive withdrawal categories. This is an oversimplification but is helpful for a brief overview. Over-reacting mood problems include anxiety conditions that lead to exaggerated fears, obsessions and worries that lead to hyper vigilance, poor concentration and poor judgment. Overactive fear leads to gross distortions of relative minor events which then threaten the stability of important relationships, job security and many routine activities. The fear of rejection may lead to a fear of isolation that may lead to a fear of a fundamental flaw within. A character flaw can then become a misplaced identity, which is much harder to repair than an insult or unfair criticism. Considering ourselves a victim of a disease instead of a good person with an illness creates a barrier to healing.

Underactive emotional expression is most often recognized as a form of depression. This is probably the most common mood disorder of our times. It involves a retreat into smaller parts of ourselves usually as a result of self-criticism and guilt or disappointment and loss of some kind. There is often an overreaction to outer events that trigger a diminished sense of self.

Excessive anger also sets in motion a wide range of reactions within us. It attracts many other attack feelings that lead to active rejection of others and self. Anger may be part of the cause of the rising epidemic of autoimmune disease. Anger diminishes our capacity to work things through because we become obsessed with eliminating the threat we feel. Large amounts of anger also attracts memories of similar situations that strengthen the need to attack or flee. Sustained anger consumes huge amounts of energy and limits the capacity to access resources for protection, understanding and eventual healing. At times intense feelings of rejection are necessary but misplaced anger may set in motion serious mood and physical disruption.

The original cause of distress is often difficult to track down and is generally not necessary for positive treatment results. The more we think the cause is another individual or group, the less likely we are identifying the true source of it until we know ourselves well. However the more we withdraw from the life around us, the less stimulation and understanding occurs within us. The more we belittle who we are the slower we grow and the more difficult it is to rise above our challenges. The initial stages of recovery require the willingness to increase our expressiveness to reactivate the higher emotions within us. These include the expressions of kindness, gratitude and goodwill, as well as calmness, confidence and cheerfulness. All of these are part of the emotional makeup of each of us, though in varying degrees of development.

The Missing Mind Matters

The mind has more to do with our basic identity and the basic roles we play in life. How we perceive the value of our family and friends has a major impact on our risk for disease. The more socially active we are, the generally greater degree of optimism. The more optimism we have, the greater sense of enjoyment of living and the less disease and distress we experience.

The mind also plays a role in how we determine our mission in life. The greater the mission the less likely we are encumbered by disease. Although disease may occur at the same incidence, or even more in some with a high mission, those with a high sense of dedication are less likely to allow it to interfere.

There are many exceptions to such general statements. However, the less sense of a mission or cherished priority the greater risk of disease. This should be considered a major cause of some problems, especially certain mood disorders.

Of course there are many who are overzealous in their missions in life whether for family or work situations. Becoming overly consumed can create imbalances that lead to depletion states, physically and emotionally. Overwork and over-anxiety often leads to poor nutrition and insomnia, both of which are essential means of maintenance and self-renewal. Often exaggerated efforts eventually force us to reevaluate our priorities that can re-start a healing effect and better balance of attention. How we use our mind determines the focus of energy of mind, heart and body. Our constant challenges slowly force us to learn better uses of mind power. As we think so we become.

The major causes of mental disease are complex but often involve a lack of development and subsequent lack of access to the tools of the mind. The basic tools of the mind are remembering, organizing, planning, analyzing and synthesizing. The most important tool is common sense: figuring out what is the basic message of this or that event or person and what to do about it. Common sense helps us establish our priorities and keeps us focused on them. Being goal-oriented helps us do so. Without goals we often flounder and get pulled in many directions, leading to frustration, confusion and lack of resolution. Just setting aside time to think things through helps keep the tools of the mind in play. Often a cause of much distress is not setting aside time to review what is happening and access our memory banks of how we have solved similar situations in the past. Deciding our ideals may be the healthiest use of the mind.

Ultimate Causes of Disease

Most diseases are connected to how we lead our daily lives. Many of the daily decisions are based on patterns of routines established for a variety of reasons over a period of time. These deserve the most attention for exploring causes of disease and distress. Major efforts to clean up our routines and be sure they represent the best we can do will prevent much distress.

One of the most obvious tendencies for disease is the family in which we are born, our gene pool of inheritance. Why are we born with certain genetic tendencies? The ultimate answer is not as important as the practical answer: if these are the circumstances, how can I best handle them? Whether it involves allergies and asthma, intestinal distress or chronic back pain, the main focus should be what can be done about it to lessen the problem, not the cause.

Gene studies are now providing the opportunity to know genetic predispositions. Samples of nuclear proteins (snips) are becoming increasingly available. If such testing leads to greater motivation for self care in preventing heart disease or cancer, disease may be more controllable. A simple version of genetic predisposition is to review the family tree of illness over the last three generations. This will provide a profile that outlines tendencies in most family members. It is always worth remembering that the family gene pool is only a tendency, and there is always room for minimizing disease and maximizing the lifestyle choices we make day in and day out.

Ultimate causes of disease involve the health of food, soil, water and air we breathe. These all affect the quality of nutrient value and possible presence of toxic matter. Even though each of these is far from perfect many of us still have options from which to choose. Organically grown food and free-range animals are generally healthier than those that are not. Filtered and purified water is better than that which is not. Walking or exercising in the country is better than doing so next to a busy vehicle area. The planet is imperfect and so too the food we grow and the animals we consume. However, vast improvements are being made over time and far less disease is caused by the environment than used to be.

Ultimate causes include the groups to which we belong. The family in which we are raised has imperfections, not only in the genes but in the habits of eating, feeling and thinking. These must be considered as we explore ourselves and the causes of our physical and psychological problems. The purpose of such a review is not to blame as much as to expand our awareness and broaden our understanding. The broader the perspective the more room there is to embrace who we are with whatever imperfections and unknowns there are.

The task to heal ultimate causes is to love ourselves more deeply, the higher nature of ourselves and the life around us. The hope and goal of most of us is to improve ourselves in every way possible. Sometimes our love has to be much deeper than we ever considered. Stretching it into the deep past is helpful at times. Healing deep causes of serious physical and psychological problems and patterns requires concerted effort over long periods of time, often with the help of professionals and trained personnel. If we are willing, healing occurs. Even if only improving slowly, moving in the right direction is deeply reassuring. We are all in it for the long haul.

Ultimate causes of disease may include the role of past lives. I have no ability to diagnose such a problem but have had my own experiences and am aware of many others' experiences. I am acquainted with those who are skilled in assessing the past to know that it has an influence on our current life. At times hearing or experiencing such a connection can be very reassuring even if deeply embarrassing. Learning the truth precedes most full healing. Being curious and interested and asking direct questions of ourself and one who may know more, is a starting point for many. Finding those with the proper training and skill can be very helpful in awakening our own self-reflection capacity.

An excellent standard upon which to draw for such a field of inquiry is the work of Edgar Cayce. He was a photographer of modest means who lived from 1877-1945. He was raised in traditional Baptist South. It was a simple life in some ways. He was very dedicated to reading the Bible, teaching Sunday school and raising a family. Through a series of events he uncovered the capacity to enter into deep trance and explore past lives of individuals requesting help. A great deal of research by many professionals has revealed a high degree of consistency and integrity in the experiences reported by him.

One of the stories from Edgar Cayce involves a woman who developed a difficult case of sexually transmitted disease. In her life reading he said that in a prior lifetime she lived in a country where she transmitted the same disease to a number of others. In this lifetime she started with a vulnerability because of her previous disregard of others and, unfortunately, activated a specific sequence of disease. Some diseases are connected in this way and require a deeper sense of willingness to forgive self and a greater regard for the precious gift of life and health we have.

Another compelling story from Cayce involves a physical therapist, Harold Reilly. Cayce referred many people to him over the years before ever meeting him. His inner guidance said that Harold was the best physical therapist in the New York City area. After they did meet and he requested a life reading from Mr. Cayce, a series of prior lifetimes was discussed. Apparently this recent series of 43 lifetimes began in the Roman times. Harold was a very successful gladiator. His error was not in performing well at that time but in pouring himself into it and loving it, of not only beating his competitors but killing them. Forty-two lifetimes later, dedicated to repairing injured bodies, he has developed great healing skill plus a high regard and reverence for the life of each of those he serves.

Over several lifetimes we have many opportunities to grow and learn, to get it right, to repair relationships and slowly bring forth the blossom of our innate beauty, joy and wisdom.

The ultimate cause of most of our problems is the lack of virtue, skill and strength. We are all working on the development of a variety of virtues from kindness to goodwill to graciousness. We identify the ones we need by the challenges we face. If we are easily discouraged the virtue we need is persistence or patience. If we are easy to anger we need to cultivate respect and tolerance for others. If we are too passive and timid, we may need courage, determination and a greater willingness to reach out, to take the initiative in meeting others and confronting problems. If we are controlling and always need to be in charge, we need more kindness and compassion for others. If we are too intellectual, we need more sense of the beauty and harmony within and around us. If we are easily caught up in unexpected distress, we need more reassurance in our deeper self and its trust in us to do the right thing in the right way. All of us need more connection to the larger whole of which we are a part so we may better draw upon its support and strength for the challenges that we face.

Expressing these virtues when needed slowly increases our skill in using them. As the skill of each unfolds we tap into the strength behind them and can call them forth with greater effect in ourselves and others.

When Not to Look For The Cause

Knowing causes of disease and distress are not necessary to know how to heal. Many steps can be taken long before we know the cause. Most of the time modern medicine is unable to describe in great depth the cause of disease, even when serious and life threatening. The focus is strongly on physical agents of disease rather than the wider spectrum of toxic energies in the earth as well as the subtle ones of thought and feeling. On the whole physicians do well enough to relieve some of the suffering and at times successfully reverse the problem than identify the cause.

Looking for the cause can be an excuse to not do the healing. I see patients at times who are obsessed with finding the cause of their problems. Needing to know the "why" can become an obstacle to healing the problem. Aspirin worked without us knowing how for many years. We can heal without knowing why and how we became ill. Children can learn how to be polite and civil without understanding the full reasons why it is needed.

Waiting to find the ultimate cause should not distract us from acting on what we know to be helpful. Why a floor is dirty or our clothes are stained is not as important as proceeding to clean them. There are always options to improve diet, exercise and attitude. Many sources of healing are always available in spite of not knowing the cause. The more we apply action to what we know, the more we learn, grow and heal. The whys and wherefores slowly unfold as we apply what we know.

Chapter 2

Activate Practical Principles of Healing

A major key to healing is the awareness that healing begins within. There is a physician within each of us that knows the source of the problem, the steps that led to it and how to work our way through it. The inner being is intelligent, wise and loving. It wants us to be well but the journey of life has obstacles along the way. Our task is to learn how to ask the right questions of ourselves to access a coherent picture of our situation and correct it. We need to learn how to find the steps that led us to where we are, identify the major turning points, the dots along the way, how to connect them and where to go from here. Over time the expanded picture unfolds and we see the grander vision of the larger whole.

Fortunately there are basic principles of healing that can show us the way. There is a map with a destination and various routes that can be taken to get us there. The journey to full health has signposts of when to go, when to stop, when to speed up and when to slow down. Too many of us identify signposts of where not to go. Many negative experiences become neon signs of distress, turmoil and despair. These need to be worked through. But there are also many points of kindness, light- heartedness, and reassuring appreciation. Exploring these is more likely to lead us toward other sources of measurable meaning and wholeness. These energies increase the healing awareness we need.

The destination of healing is whole health of body, heart, and mind. Most of us seek just to have a healthy body forgetting that the body is sick because of the decisions made or not made by the heart and mind. In fact we are a larger presence of life than the physical frame and its many marvelous organs and cells. We need to appreciate the five wonderful senses of sight, sound, taste, smell and touch but also move beyond them.

Surrendering the things of youth gracefully is not a common occurrence. For many, the goal is a thinner body, a taller body and one with more energy. Many dread to get on the scale because of what they will see. Even normal weight women often feel too heavy and too short. Men are less concerned about the body appearance but do not want to admit they have a problem. I often see men who want an exam and deny any significant problem until I ask directly about each part of the body. After that it is apparent more than a few conditions are present and some require serious attention. When real physical problems are present there is often little awareness into the connections with stressful changes in a major relationship at home or work.

The basic principles of healing can be learned to reverse most problems and prevent further ones. When pursued regularly we can enable a more free flow of healing energy that increases vitality and greater function. The first goal of healing is to align ourselves with the source of healing, the higher self. In turn its influence awakens the higher mind to an intelligent focus with practical problem solving. Then the energy of the mind can expand the heart toward hopefulness, enthusiasm and optimism. These in turn bathe the body with a fresh flow of healing energy.

The Capacity To Heal Is Always With Us

The source of healing is always with us. It is part of the essence of who we are. It is like the sun that shines upon us. Even during cloudy days it is our source of warmth, light and life. Like the sun our source of healing continuously sends the energy of vitality, self-renewal and repair ability. In spite of clouds of fear and worry energy moves from the higher realms of our being to the mind, heart and body. Our essential nature at its core includes many attributes of healing such as goodwill, tolerance, forgiveness, integrity, patience, persistence, and wholeness. Each of these contributes to the ability to be well and stay well. The energy of healing is a multi-dimensional department that draws upon many inner strengths of character. At first there are only glimpses of these strengths. As we heal the clouds of doubt and despair so too does our healing presence expand and function in more effective ways.

We are born with the capacity to heal. Physically, healing starts at an early age because we need it to survive. Colostrum is the first few days of mother's milk for breastfeeding; it is filled with antibodies, downloaded from the mother to the infant. Within a few months and with exposures, the immune system quickly builds itself to eventually fight a wide range of bacteria, viruses and fungi. The plant and animal kingdoms have been evolving protective chemicals over long periods of time. A varied diet helps to transfer this experience into our bodies. The greater the health of our diet and exercise routine the healthier is the immune system's ability to prevent disease and reverse it when necessary.

The full function of our immune system depends to some extent on what we inherit. There are some differences, most noticeable in those with allergy tendencies, chronic pain, intestinal ills, hormone conditions and increased risk for certain tumors. However, lifestyle patterns will enhance or diminish the inherited immune system functions depending on the extent to which we pursue them.

We are also born with an ability to heal emotional and mental problems. There are built-in capacities to handle psychological stresses and disruptions. Within each of us is varying degrees of wellbeing, defenses and abilities to heal distress. Our basic psychological immunity consists of understanding, insight, meaning and the ability to act on them. These energy forces enable us to recover from perceived and real personal stress, learn from experiences of life and insulate us from unnecessary harm of them. We may also become deeply deficient if overusing the resources we have.

Our ability to heal is part of who we are from the time we are born. We come with instructions built in. However, there must be a genuine interest in learning how to use this ability and awaken its full potential for helping us. We must be willing to set aside the time to read, study and cooperate with it. We do this by observing how life affects us, the people with whom we interact, circumstances we encounter and reactions we generate.

Healing energy is always present. It is up to us find its sources and how to activate it. Just as we have air, water and food available to us in more than sufficient quantity, we still need to learn how to identify clean, healthy sources of them, how to access them, prepare them for use and do so on a regular, consistent basis. The sources of healing are present in our spirit, mind, heart and body but awaits our capacity to access and mobilize them effectively.

Healing Is Always Occurring

As long as we are alive, healing is occurring. Healing is most rapid and effective when young but readily awakened every day of life, especially when triggered by injury or infection. It is said that there is an average of 70 infections in each of us at any given time. I'm sure most of these must be on the skin, mouth and nose. But we certainly must have an active immune system to survive for even short periods of time. The body is learning how to mobilize healing from day one with many peaks and valleys along the way.

It should be noted that every organ of the body participates in healing. Each organ has its own specially designed immune cells. The nose, throat and sinuses have their team, as do the lungs, the intestines, the muscles and the brain. Especially at night the healing members swing into full action, exploring every nook and cranny for weaknesses and invaders of any kind. During this time nutrients are distributed to every organ and cell of the body, especially the areas in greatest need to optimize function and repair disruption. The greater the health of each organ, the greater the resilience and capacity of the body as a whole for full recovery from illness.

Psychologically we are always reviewing, processing and integrating the experiences of the day. Like the news of the day, there is an ongoing gathering of events large and small. And while the events unfold around us, a swirl of feeling is stirred up within us. Our most recent interactions, feelings and thoughts are continuously being interwoven with our database of emotions, memories and habits. Routine activities occur that do not need special attention. Frequently more must be done. Triggers of fear, doubt and worry will attract memories of the same, especially of unresolved issues. Every interaction is fit into who we are. What doesn't fit must be shaped and molded or set aside for a later time. Although it is true that problems worsen as we focus on them, connections are also being made with the prior experiences of solving the problems we've had.

Our family and friends are often ready sources of positive perspectives. They remind us of the pleasure of our company, the enjoyment of shared activities and ready willingness to overlook poor decisions and clumsy interactions. So, too, the inner storage of thoughts and feelings have many memories of how to reassure us in times of turmoil and how to consider fair and unfair criticism. Most of all, healing occurs as we learn from the mistakes we make and the suffering we go through.

Healing energy is closely aligned with the energy of learning and growing. As we learn and grow we increase access to the energy of healing. To the extent that we are awake and alert, observing what happens in us and around us, we are slowly expanding. With every new event and interaction with people and circumstances we are increasing our capacity for receiving healing energy.

There Are Many Obstacles To Healing

There are many obstacles to healing for each of us. These can be found in the way we use our body, our emotions, our mind and spirit. Although healing energy is always present and flowing, we can limit its effect by the choices we make or fail to make.

Most of the common physical obstacles to healing are apparent to us as the presence of unhealthy habits and the lack of healthy ones. The habits of over-consuming alcohol, tobacco and sugar strains specific organs of the body and diminishes their contribution to the health of the body. Over eating leads to many diseases of excess weight including hyperglycemia, diabetes, knee pain, hip pain and back pain. A poor diet over time can lead to micronutrient malnutrition, in turn leading to triggering or worsening the common diseases of fatigue, arthritis, allergies, autoimmune and heart disease. Insufficient exercise leads to decreased strength, stamina, muscle stiffness and pain. Over-exercise causes muscle strain, infection and heart disease. Inadequate sleep diminishes alertness, memory and vitality, essential elements for a full, active day. Oversleep is a sign of depletion of organ vitality or depression of mood.

Chronic disease is a common obstacle. We get used to the illness, consider it chronic and begin to believe it will be with us always. We wait for it to go away, consult one or more physicians or health practitioners with limited success and then see it as a constant companion.

The least hint that a problem is genetic can easily become a barrier to healing. If it is in the genes it will not change. This is not true, but there is a strong set of beliefs that our core source of cell growth does not change much over time, that the gene structure is set in stone. Thus, allergies, hypertension, weight gain, headaches, low back pain and a host of other potentially genetic conditions become seen as intractable.

Failing to see improvement is an obstacle to healing. Overeating is the most common form of perceived failure. Most people overweight have been on several diets. There is usually partial success, occasionally dramatic. However, most people also put weight back on. I worked at a spa retreat center for several years. A major draw to the center was the fasting program, the main use of which was for those wanting to lose weight. All succeeded in part, some more than others. Over time many returned to the program and occasionally we did a survey of how people maintained the progress gained while with us. Some continued the improvement over a year later, however most gained back much or all the weight. Many other benefits were learned in the process but often the chronicity of being overweight itself becomes a barrier to healing. If several good efforts don't work well enough, is it possible to succeed?

Alcohol and drugs have much worse consequences to health and longevity than overweight. They have more impact on the chemistry of the brain, which controls behavior patterns. When the nerve hormones are trained to fire in response to what we eat, drink, ingest or inject we develop strong habits that are hard to break. Compelling habits create channels of energy in specific directions limiting where else energy can flow. Like a deep rut in a road prevents the car from going near it, so too does strong negative habits prevent healthier habits from forming. If most of our ways of living are feeding certain bad habits there is less energy available for new healthy habits however well intentioned or desired.

Getting discouraged too easily is a common obstacle. We often start with good intention, especially with apparent results. But too many of us give up too quickly. Asking for help is often a good idea, but when we do not see better results from further input there is a tendency to get discouraged and stop looking. Instead of reassessing the reasons why advice from others doesn't work many give up and get depressed. Decisions to shut down diminish new incentives and new possibilities. Over time it can lead to serious depression. It is deadly to not want to change.

The types of people with whom we associate may become obstacles to health and healing. There are those who will encourage us to drink, smoke or gamble. Others have habits of fear, anger, blaming and complaining. All of these should be considered obstacles to optimal health and healing energy. "Misery loves company" is a truism that predates Shakespeare. As we feed off other people's stories of dismay and delay we gather more excuses to stay the way we are, which is usually a downward spiral. Nothing ever stays the way it is. Eventually inertia can become as big as a mountain of immovable stone as the problem itself.

Habits of negative emotions are obstacles to healing. Common emotional obstacles to healing are that we may be too easily overwhelmed and full of fear, worry, grief or anger. Our emotions are magnets that attract energy of its kind. Just as the magnet becomes cluttered with a disordered array of metal pieces, we may have clusters of fears, frustrations and worries. They not only are unpleasant to see and feel, they can foul our basic mood and sense of well-being. Feelings of fear diminish expressions of confidence to follow directions to heal and establish better habits of health in body and mind. Worry diminishes our sense of serenity and calmness. It often leads to over-reacting to events and important people in our life, often making things worse than they were. Anger intensifies our rejection of others and ourselves when we most need them. Grief deters gratitude and gracefulness instead of helping us adapt to loss and learn from it.

Denial is an obstacle to healing. The most common form of fear is denial. Until we recognize a problem we are not going to seek help correcting it. The value in denial is that it protects us from fear and consequences. Men who have a heart attack and deny the severity of it have fewer immediate complications of it than those who worry and dread the effects of it. They leave the hospital sooner but die earlier. Denial is only a temporary fix, like a Band-Aid over a serious wound. The underlying problem will fester further until addressed.

When I was going through medical training I remember a patient of my teacher. The latest tests showed that her colon cancer had spread leaving her with a poor prognosis for living much longer. And yet her physician did not explain the seriousness of her condition revealed by the tests. When I asked him why he didn't inform his patient about her current status, he took me back into the room of the patient and asked her how much she would like to know about her condition. It became quite apparent she didn't want to know the truth and would live her life as long as she could until the end. Denial is a powerful defense of suffering but only postpones the truth and the real path to healing.

I met one fellow who came to me for alternative treatments for a tumor on his neck. It was obviously large when I saw him the first time. He had recently received a diagnosis of cancer of the tonsil. However, he first noticed a small lump in the area seven years before, thinking it was due to a vehicle accident. He kept thinking it would go away and avoided treatment for several years. Denial diminishes our interest in finding options of healing.

Anger is a serious barrier to healing. It has several forms besides the overt display of a temper tantrum. More commonly is the expression to a friend or family of bitter complaint about someone or something in their life. When fostered and fussed over and over it ferments and festers into a serious infection of the mood. It often makes us much worse than the one we blame and complain about.

Several years ago many studies were performed around the concept of types of personality. Type A was considered to be vigilant, time-oriented, impulsive and driven. They became known as the "worried well," not overtly ill but often anxious about themselves and their life. Type B people were considered to be more relaxed, easy-going, flexible and less driven to perform. Type A's tended to be worriers and a bit more susceptible to certain diseases compared to Type B's seemed calmer, though still susceptible to certain other problems. Type A folks were found to be more susceptible to heart disease, especially early heart attacks and strokes. The studies were not strongly conclusive until Type A's were broken down into four categories. The worst category Type A most susceptible to serious heart disease early in life was found to be those who were most likely hostile, angry and impulsive.

Anger is especially detrimental when applied to self as a reaction to something embarrassing or fearful. It is not only an expression of rejection but also a desire to destroy and eliminate. Although varying with the intensity, it always has a negative effect on the flow of healing resources within us. Anger should not be mistaken for a strong, determined, honest expression of integrity confronting a difficult situation or person. A firm, even loud expression of strength or courage for a good cause is not anger. Anger is an expression of annoyance for a self-serving cause. It is often complaining to protect self without participating in solving or healing the issue at hand.

Grief may be an obstacle to healing. Compassion is a virtue among those caring for the dying. It is an instinct to feel sorrow for what is missing, especially close family and friends on whom we relied for enjoyment, sympathy, acceptance, goodwill and generosity. However, prolonged sorrow disconnects us from the good that we continue to receive from those who have passed on. Overly indulging grief clouds the connection to our higher self that wants us to identify the value of the relationship and honor it by increasing our own expression of it. Every loss of any kind is an opportunity to learn detachment from the form nature of our loss to the beauty and strength of what has been gained in the relationship.

A lack of interest in learning is an obstacle to healing. The mind is especially designed to be curious and interested in learning with a sense of adventure and a spirit of exploration. A young child is naturally this way, often passing through a phase of wanting to know why and how to everything it sees. For many reasons there is a tendency to lose these instincts and not develop them into skills. Trauma, rejection, stress and a host of events can lead to false conclusions and the accumulation of negative uses of the mind. A lack of curiosity is an obstacle to healing because without it we limit our learning and become more subject to isolation. We insulate ourselves from the immense array of new ideas and opportunities around us.

Overuse of the mind can be an obstacle. If given too much power fault-finding will only increase our ability to tear down and destroy. At times celebrities act with authority outside their area of expertise. Authorities without real knowledge and skill are like the emperor without clothes, espousing untruths and generalities that expose more about what they don't know than what they do. We must monitor ourselves at times and not over extend what we do know into realms that we don't have much awareness. Obsessions with certain issues of people and politics can distract us from a balanced use of our attention and energy. It has been suggested that the intensity of religion has been transferred to politics for many, to their detriment. This especially applies to obsessions with personal issues as well.

There is a role for a critical mind, authoritative decision-making and truth. However overuses of knowing what is wrong or not working is an obstacle to healing. A high degree of conscience is necessary for healing but a strong inner critic will grind us under. A homegrown inner tyrant or terrorist can cause serious damage to our self-esteem and self-concept. Unhealthy authority needs to be exposed and expelled.

The goal of the healthy mind is to reveal the plan of growth, direction and expression of the inner being, so that we manifest the contribution of our highest calling. Whatever inhibits, distracts or distorts this goal is an obstruction and eventually must be overcome. This is done by reaching for, calling forth and expressing the higher nature of our being.

There Are Many Ways To Remove The Obstacles To Healing

To grow and change is essential to healing. Do you want to be comfortable or do you want to change? To grow healthy plants we have to provide healthy soil, water and some light. To keep growing the plants we must change the soil or add fertilizer to replenish the nutrients available. As long as we are awake and alive we have the capacity to choose to change or stay the way we are. As we exercise our choices of the day from small to large, we grow in our ability to effect the changes needed and desired. The more we choose healthy foods to eat the easier it is to do so. The foods for the mind of healing are sincerity, devotion and truth.

Sincerity is the heart of healing. The 12 step alcoholics anonymous program is an exceptional program to develop honesty and sincerity. It represents a basic set of principles that are simple, succinct and readily usable. It begins with a genuine call for help, a sincere appeal for support from the life within, the higher power, the source of our true self. A declaration of need mobilizes the strength of sincerity we have to admit the problem and prepare a plan for addressing it. We clarify the basic need to be healthy by sincerely identifying how being healthy serves us, those who rely on us and the obligations we have incurred.

A heartfelt sense of devotion to greater health draws forth new habits to replace the old ones that are expiring. Just as flowers go through stages from bulb to blossom to a natural end, so too habits begin small, grow slowly, mature to a full size, then begin to die. With human habits we must choose to change. Habits form a life of their own even when destructive. The best of habits outlive their purpose in time. Dedicated devotion calls forth a heartfelt commitment to accept the point of health we have and build upon it. It supports our efforts to pour ourselves into this stage of health, plan on the next steps to take and pursue them diligently.

Truth is the antidote to denial and ignorance. Awakening the need to know the full truth of this illness, this habit or this dysfunction increases the capacity to understand it and come up with a plan to overcome it. Truth has power. It connects us to a greater use of the mind to find the reasons why we need to be well. The more reasons we have to be well the more mind power we bring to the table. The more mind power at the table the more options from which to choose and the energy that comes with them. Pursuing the truth of who we are can be a path from the obvious to the abstract to the subtle beauties of life. The practical truth is to identify the problem and the resources we have to face it.

Mobilize Healing Directly

Direct healing is the straight appeal to the higher self for healing. At times, healing is accelerated by a sincere strong appeal to the higher self. The higher self can hasten healing with focused intensity and determination.

Inspired insight is a clear understanding of the cause of the problem. Often we get confused and simply don't think things through. We give up too easily and allow problems to grow until a crisis occurs before making new decisions. We think the problem is the diagnosis of the illness, the pain, the fatigue or the depression. There is a strong tendency to identify the problem with the physical presence of it, diminishing or excluding the role of the emotions, mind and personality.

Insight leads us to the true cause. A diagnosis of the illness is often helpful in treating acute problems and many chronic, severe problems. But it is rarely sufficient to heal the problem. Insight detaches us from irrelevant issues and comments of others.

When working at the Pain Clinic we had a patient with chronic low back pain. It began when he was bending over to fix the battery in an airplane. He worked for a large airline company and was one of three engineers in the repair crew for one hangar. The least favorite task was to repair the battery of an aircraft. They are heavy, hard to move and very time consuming. As the batteries were not getting done on schedule the supervisor finally required them to rotate the task. Eventually it became my patient's responsibility because the other two left it for him to do. He detested doing the job but let the others defer it to him.

While with us he developed insight of the cause of his back pain. His timid side caused him to slip into an unfair responsibility that he came to resent. His subconscious took him out of the conflict but at the cost of chronic back pain. As he regained a greater sense of confidence he confronted his timidness, forgave himself and healed remarkably well.

Dynamic determination is a concerted effort to start a new program for healing ourselves. I have a patient with a history of drug and alcohol abuse. He has had chronic back pain that led to many doctors, prescriptions and then alcohol. Over time he accepted the fact that the drugs and alcohol were a separate problem, an additional disease making his life more complicated and depressing. He began to ask for help, attend meetings and avoid people who were abusing drugs and alcohol. Eventually he overcame both problems, had surgeries to correct most of the ailments he suffered and reentered the profession he had chosen.

A new sense of persistence can mobilize a new surge of intention. Often that includes other people. There is no question that more people lose weight when in a group program to do so. This doesn't mean we are relying on others to do our job. It means that our new effort is willing to access the full breadth of support available to us including the learning and help from others. Such a greater willingness usually leads to a greater receptiveness to our own inner resources as well, the memories of the many ways we've helped ourselves and those who have given us the example to do so. Our inner resources for greater dedication to heal are immense but must be mobilized to have an impact.

Regenerate Physical Well Being

Chapter 3

Five Steps to Nutrient Excellence

Basic benefits of nutrition include many obvious ones and many that are not often recognized. The most obvious benefit is to provide energy. A good diet provides energy by increasing the prevalence of building blocks for new cell growth, repair and maintenance. Each of these activities ensures optimal organ function and general vitality. If functioning well we have the energy we need for the day's activities, the relationship interactions and the work we have to do. We recover normally from most illnesses and injuries. We have the energy and interest in pursuing the tasks and challenges of the day however routine, difficult or unusual they may be. We have the energy to help where needed, to recognize people and groups worth serving and doing our part to advance their cause.

Vitality and cell upkeep require a wide range of nutrients, commonly separated into macro- and micronutrients. The macronutrients are the proteins, carbohydrates and fats. The micronutrients are the vitamins, minerals, and diverse combinations of these.

The macronutrients have healthy and unhealthy types of proteins, carbohydrates and fats. There are essential and nonessential types of each of these. We need optimal amounts of each for a dynamic, healthy body. The best kinds of protein are the fish and fowl, though vegetable sources may be adequate for some. The best fats are found in sufficient supply in vegetables.

The best carbohydrates are found in vegetables and most fruits. Grains have modest amounts of proteins, carbohydrates and few oils, but they are not an essential food group unless other options are limited.

The micronutrients depend on the quality and variety of foods eaten. If we eat well we should not need supplements for micronutrients. However life is complicated by family history, age, injury, illness, stress and how food is grown. As a result requirements for a wide range of micronutrients increases in a variety of ways. Ideally blood, urine and saliva specimen testing would reveal our optimal needs. Even though cutting edge testing is available and useful, results may not be individualized enough for high level wellness. The simplest solution may be a good multivitamin that even research scientists are now recommending.

What Is The Best Diet For Healthy Well Being?

This is the question we all need to ask ourselves at some point in our busy lives. What is the best diet for healthy living, full energy for the day, disease prevention and rapid recovery from injury or illness? This can vary widely but general suggestions can be given. Basically there must be adequate protein and healthy amounts of essential carbohydrates and fats.

Proteins provide the basic structure for all the organs, muscles, nerves, bones and hormones. They are a major source of energy and repair material to help us recover from a wide variety of illness and injury. The best sources are fish and fowl because of ease of digestion and minimal fat content. Lean meats from beef and pork are protein rich and excellent for many but are not the best source for some. Vegetables and grains may provide a sufficient amount of protein in the right combinations. Powder proteins work for many and may be necessary for some. The amounts of protein needed vary widely and can be measured by blood tests, energy level and individual satisfaction.

Carbohydrates provide the main source of quick energy. They are often easily broken down into sugars which can be readily used by the brain and other organs. The various types of carbohydrates are best provided by vegetables because they are also rich in anti-oxidants and multiple phyto nutrients.

Raw is better than cooked if they are sufficiently digestible. The fiber rich content of raw vegetables helps to ensure slow absorption limiting weight gain and blood sugar elevations. Raw foods also ensure bulk residue for intestinal function and elimination preventing constipation and congestion. The best vegetables are those that grow above the ground since they have less risk for starch excess and subsequent weight gain. Five to seven half-cup servings per day is an excellent amount.

Fats are necessary for all cell membrane function and nerve conduction. The outer lining of cells protects them from environmental toxins, viruses and bacteria. The membranes of nerve cells facilitate conduction and communication to and from all parts of the body. Essential fats contribute to healing injured tissue by initially inflaming injured tissue to attract sufficient repair material followed by dysinflaming them to complete the recovery process. The healthiest fats are vegetable oils and olive oil. Blood tests can be done to monitor these levels.

The Best Fluid Is Water

The best fluid is always water. The benefits of adequate fluid are pervasive, and essential for every organ of the body. The respiratory, intestinal, urinary and cardiovascular systems all function well with full water fluid amounts.

The mouth, sinuses and lungs perform best with high hydration levels. Their primary goal is to filter food and air to allow greater contact between immune cells and harmful viruses and bacteria. Colds and flu viruses are less likely to invade body tissues when the body has maximum moisture amounts that allow greater ease of mucus flow and cleansing immune cell mixture.

The intestinal tract requires free fluid levels to enhance healthy acid and enzyme distribution. The first step to reverse constipation is sufficient fluid amounts to ease debris discharge from food, fiber and bile residue. Good fluid levels prevent concentrations of toxins and bile from inflammatory effects on the intestinal lining cells. The solution to pollution is dilution and ease of access of the immune system at all times in all spaces.

The urinary tract filters the blood stream continuously. Through an intricate process it monitors the concentrations and types of minerals, immune substances and hormones. It allows diffusion through the filtering units that then actively reabsorb what the body needs. Optimal fluid levels prevent and treat urinary infections in women and men. Dehydration is a frequent cause of infection in the urinary, intestinal and respiratory systems.

The cardiovascular system benefits from high fluid intake by slightly thinning the blood, preventing risk for clot formation. As the body ages, sluggish blood flow in the tiny vessels of the heart and brain are at less risk for disease conditions with smoother fluid flow and an optimal hydration level.

Sodas, smoothies, juice, coffee and alcohol are best consumed at very modest levels. If weight or blood sugar levels are too high, total restriction of sodas, smoothies and juice is essential for success. Coffee and alcohol are actually helpful to many, although more than modest amounts may lead to serious problems with the intestines, liver, brain and heart. Indigestion, anxiety and heart irregularities are at times triggered by excess amounts of caffeine.

Water is the best liquid. Even weight loss can be aided by sufficient fluid amounts that increase the sense of fullness before and during a meal. Optimal amounts are 6-8 six-ounce glasses per day. As the quality of water is of growing concern, filtered, ozone and bottled water are in growing demand. For those concerned about increasing amounts of toxic minerals and chemicals in the water supply, hair and urine analyses can be performed.

Organic Versus Inorganic Foods

Foods grown with healthy fertilizer have more nutrients than those without. In the Midwest it has been known for years that grains with optimal fertilizing have up to 30% higher protein levels in some fields. Mineral levels are also optimal in organic foods that may be important in older people. As we age we don't efficiently extract needed nutrients from the foods we eat and thereby unknowingly create clinical deficiencies. Range-fed beef, pork and dairy have higher concentrations of essential omega fatty acids. These fats are found in the natural food chain, not the commercial cage or stall grain-fed animals. Frozen vegetables are generally very healthy. Homegrown vegetables and fruits are the healthiest and most nutrient-packed if given good care. They are best when picked mature with maximum nutrient content. Commercial foods are often harvested early so they do not over-ripen before purchase and consumption.

Foods To Minimize Or Avoid

Processed foods, sugars and animal products are the main foods to minimize or eliminate from your diet. Processed grains have many fewer vitamins, minerals and proteins than the most natural, raw forms. Of course processing is done for the purpose of delaying spoiling and continues to serve many without readily available fresh food sources. The extent to which we can choose fresh foods should always be maximized.

Sugars have dramatically increased in the food chain. In the last 50 years the high amounts of sugar have led to epidemics of overweight, obesity and diabetes. The primary source of sugar has been soda, however the penetration of sugar into common foods also continues to rise. Ketchup, toothpaste, and canned foods are often filled with sugar.

Disease conditions from excess sugar have created an epidemic of diabetes. Even mild elevations of glucose in the blood increase the disease conditions of diabetes. There is increased weight that leads to increased wearing of back, hip and knee joints. Increased blood sugar increases arteriosclerosis that in turn leads to earlier heart disease, kidney insufficiency and skin atrophy. Nerve degeneration leading to neuropathies, memory loss and Alzheimer's syndrome is accelerated by diabetes and hyperglycemia. There is increased risk for infections in the respiratory tract, urinary system and skin.

Hypoglycemia is also a disease. It became a very popular disease 40 years ago. Blood sugar levels that dip too low can result in headaches, dizziness and fainting. Pain, fatigue and decreased thinking can all contribute to less than optimal function until corrected. Hypoglycemia sometimes is a precursor to hyperglycemia. It is possible that the hypoglycemic epidemic years ago preceded the diabetes epidemic. Although there are many treatment suggestions for hypoglycemia, the simple ones are consuming more consistent protein three times a day and decreasing refined sugar ingestion.

Gluten allergy is finally receiving the attention it deserves. I first learned about gluten-caused conditions over 30 years ago. My colleague physician, mentor and friend, Dr. Evarts Loomis, who founded the Meadowlark Retreat Center, became healthier and more energetic when avoiding gluten products. He was primarily of English heritage. The English and Irish are especially prone to this food reaction because the growing of gluten grains did not begin there until about 1,000 years ago. In the European and Asian countries it began over 10,000 years ago allowing a more complete DNA digestive enzyme evolution to develop. The digestive enzyme system has many ways it can specialize and does so over long periods of time. It is the incomplete digestion of the gluten products that leads to an immune reaction and subsequent inflammation of multiple organ systems.

Gluten sensitivity, apart from gluten allergy, is a recognized condition among a growing number of research gastroenterologists. It can also lead to intestinal symptoms of nausea, heartburn, diarrhea and cramping. It can affect the brain and nervous system interfering with sleep, mood and cognitive capacity. It can affect the skin, muscle strength and energy level. Incompletely processed foods affect every organ of the body and their many functions.

Gluten is found in all the grains, especially wheat, barley, rye, couscous and semolina. Oats may contain gluten although some are gluten-free. Rice is the safest grain. A celiac blood screen can be done at all major labs to assess the severity of gluten immune status. A negative test means that a major gluten allergy is not present, but gluten hypersensitivity may still be present and contribute to medical conditions.

What Is The Value Of Fasting?

Fasting is one of the oldest known methods for healing and regeneration. I worked at Dr. Loomis' Meadowlark Retreat Center, a pioneering holistic health spa in Hemet, California for ten years. The main feature of the program was the fasting regimen that had three levels of fasting: only vegetables, vegetable juices and water. I participated in the fasting of over 3,000 individuals during that time. There were many dramatic improvements in physical and psychological well-being. Weight loss, decreased lipids, decreased blood sugar, decreased hypertension, decreased joint pain and clearer thinking were common benefits noted, often within a few days.

One of the most dramatic lipid changes occurred in a man with a prior total cholesterol of about 900 and triglycerides of over 1200. His blood looked like cream when it was collected. Within two weeks in the fasting program his total cholesterol came down to 350 and the triglycerides to about 400. A diabetologist in San Francisco puts all new patients on a three-day vegetable juice fast. The blood sugar level returns to normal in all of them confirming the immense role of diet in diabetes.

Vegetable juice fasting is easier to maintain for longer periods of time. Juice and water fasting should always be supervised by experienced personnel, particularly when doing it for the first time or when medical conditions are present. Blood tests, an electrocardiogram and a physical exam help to ensure adequate cardiovascular health and energy during the fast. A three-day juice fast is done by some people on a monthly basis with very positive results. For weight loss, most individuals do better finding a consistent diet they can use for an extended period of time.

Our fasting program strongly emphasized a wide range of classes for introspection and new life direction. There were classes on dream work, meditation and prayer. As a result many individuals reported inspiring insight that helped to heal the body, relationships and disappointments. The more holistic the approach the more likely major changes will occur and continue.

Weight Loss Options

More people learn about nutrition because of a need to lose weight than any other reason. The number of people overweight is now over 65% in the U.S., half of whom are obese, meaning over 20% above the ideal weight. Overweight leads to many medical conditions, often grouped together as metabolic syndrome. Besides excess weight this syndrome includes elevated cholesterol, blood pressure, and blood sugar. In addition, obesity often leads to early joint disease of the knees and hips and is now the leading cause of fatty liver dysfunction. Yet the problems of overweight are generally not enough to motivate most people to lose weight and keep it off. The essential need is to recognize the many values of being healthy. The more reasons we have to be healthy the more likely we will succeed in our efforts to do so. Each of us is a precious piece of life deserving the best of health possible to serve the highest purposes for living.

There are many ways to lose weight if followed persistently. The simplest is to avoid the obvious high calorie foods and emphasize raw vegetables and lean meats. In other words, fish and fowl for protein, raw or cooked vegetables for complex carbohydrates and vegetable oils for healthy fats. Modest amounts of chewable fruit may be acceptable like apples, persimmons and dried fruit. For many this is easier said than done.

A stronger preference to weight loss than diet is to find a supplement that works. There are many supplement options that can help lose weight. I am not aware of any of them having a consistent effect on a large number of people except the amino acid combination of tyrosine, 5 HTP, cysteine and dopamine. This is a neurotransmitter program approach used in many weight loss programs with continued success. Essentially these are specific proteins that increase nerve energy to take the place of decreasing energy from calorie cutbacks. Neuroresearch.com is one of a growing number of online sites for this approach.

Nerve hormone programs emphasize the intake of increasing amounts of amino acids over 3-4 weeks. Many are monitored with urine testing for the hormone levels of serotonin, dopamine, noradrenaline and adrenaline. Changes are made based on the results of the testing. The right amounts of nerve hormones and precursors have a helpful influence on every organ of the body. They help optimize all the hormone sources of the body that are necessary to maintain high energy levels. Ensuring high energy supports the need for a full exercise routine in spite of decreased calorie intake. Full energy and exercise help to keep the mood stable while choosing the best foods available day by day. However, it is necessary for some to consume only 900 calories per day to lose weight on this program.

The most successful way to lose weight over a long period of time is to join a group effort. Weight loss programs are largely successful because of the group support rendered. As a group of individuals meet on a weekly basis they form a bond of reassurance, personal experience and gems of learning. Sharing small successes builds a sense of optimism that is essential to changing habits as deep as eating. Small group work helps us learn how to handle the many distractions from healthy eating. They address the big issues of how to handle holidays, birthdays and visits by family or friends. Most of all the small group of new friends encourages us to forgive ourselves more quickly when we falter and fall back from our best intentions. Guilt and depression can rob us of new efforts to do it well. Group support, enjoyment and enthusiasm help build a momentum of success that is very effective over time.

Even group efforts are not enough for many when the group disbands. Every food has thousands of chemicals that trigger many physical reactions in the body every time we eat. Certain drugs are addicting and so is food. Eating habits are part of our genetic code, driven by the deep urge to survive and thrive. If each reaction is a voice telling us what to eat next, there are many voices in the body. The solution to long-term success is establishing multiple sources of support. Family, friends and support groups can continue their good efforts when pursued consistently. The greatest allies are habits of high purpose, persistence and perseverance in spite of the many obstacles and events of living.

A major goal in eating well is to learn how to empower the knowledge we already know. The healthiest voices within us know what is best for body, heart and mind. Identifying our highest intentions for eating well helps to activate the strength of choosing well. For some this is not difficult. For many it is a lifelong struggle that is worth pursuing. Answering these questions may help access the best voices you need to hear:

1. What is the best use of the energy in the food I consume?
2. What foods do I know are best for the health of my whole self?

3. What are the sources of strength within me that I want to be in charge of the choices I make today in the foods I eat?
4. How can I remind myself what is best every time before I begin to eat?

The Wise Use Of Supplements

Supplements are playing an increasing role in the health of most Americans. Over 75% of us take supplements to some extent. Most do not discuss it with their doctor because there is low interest, low knowledge and possible criticism, although that is changing. The main reason to consider adding supplements to even a good diet is to optimize nutrient levels. Past and recent studies reveal that our nutrient value food chain has diminished over time. Healthy foods are not as healthy as we assume. The Department of Agriculture studies indicate that most nutrients are not only less than what we thought but are also decreasing if we don't choose wisely.

William Willet M.D., Ph.D. is the author of *Eat, Drink and Be Healthy*. He is a physician researcher who recommends a multivitamin for all older adults. Currently, Willett is the Fredrick John Stare Professor of Epidemiology and Nutrition and the chair of the department of nutrition at Harvard School of Public Health. He is also a professor of medicine at Harvard Medical School and has published more than 1,000 scientific articles regarding various aspects of diet and disease. He is the second most cited author in clinical medicine.

Individual needs for supplements can be measured by blood and urine tests. Genova is one of a growing number of laboratories that measure vitamin, mineral, protein and fatty acid levels with a test called Nutreval. These tests are reliable in measuring current micronutrient levels. What isn't clear is the noticeable improvement with optimizing these levels. In other words, will you be healthy with less disease and more energy if you bring all these levels to the mid- or upper-range of normal? That is not guaranteed though there are many reasons to do so.

This test and others also measure toxic heavy metals load. There is increasing interest in some circles that these play a major role in chronic disease. I have measured these levels in many patients over the years. Although the tests often show excessive amounts, corrective measures rarely reveal improvements. There are many ways to decrease heavy metal levels. Even when repeat testing shows a return to normal, healthy amounts, signs of improved health are not commonly apparent. Nonetheless, this is an area to consider, especially in those with chronic disease that is not responding to the usual conventional and alternative approaches.

The most comprehensive well-documented compendium of supplement use is called *Nutritional Medicine* by Alan Gaby, M.D. It draws upon a massive number of studies that have been done over the years on nutritional medicine and the use of supplements. It discusses over 400 health conditions with dietary and supplement suggestions with an extensive list of references for each one. I have found this source of immense value for many patients.

The other well-documented source of the use of supplements for medical conditions is *Disease Prevention and Treatment* by Life Extension. Life Extension is a supplement company that is dedicated to informing the public about the value of nutritional health. It has a monthly magazine highlighting the role of nutrition and supplements based on current research. Their mission is to "translate diverse scientific findings into therapeutic protocols that can be understood by the lay public." They are determined to review and inform the public about medical research that has practical value for the relief of pain and suffering. I have no financial investment in Life Extension.

Along with many individual supplements there are many combination remedy products. These combination products usually include the most researched supplements for the conditions intended. Some of these conditions are designed to treat hypertension, fatigue, memory loss, insomnia and osteoporosis. The downside of combination products is that the products included are often in only modest amounts and thus less likely for optimal effects.

Mind, Mood And Food

"Let food be your medicine and medicine your food" is the ancient principle of Hippocrates, the great Greek physician. He established many principles of practice that are as true now as then. He also said that nature is the great healer. The task for us is to define what is the most natural way to eat to be healthy for our own unique self. How can we attune to the essential true nature of our body, heart and mind to learn what is most needed? Do we satisfy our taste buds' desire for pleasure, our stomach's desire to be filled or our need for energy, resilience and stamina? Are we interested in the moment's need for nourishment or the long-term nutrients for healthy living and exhilarated aging?

The instinct for pleasure from food is strong, which is why there is increasing weight concerns around the world. For the first time in eons food is readily available to many. When we can have what we want, many of us choose what tastes good more often than what is good for us. So we have to learn how to restrain automatic impulses for sugar, salt and spices to prevent overweight and other problems. The first goal is to become informed about what is healthy and then establish guidelines for what is best.

Fortunately a great deal of research has been done to show us the best foods to emphasize. Knowledge helps us learn how to rise above instinct. After learning the urges of the body we need to learn the urges of the emotions. Fear, worry, guilt and anger are powerful forces that influence our choices of food. Alcohol, coffee and nicotine are obviously abused by many of us to calm down or pick us up. It is not enough to know what to eat; you need to know how to do so with the many choices available and the multiple moods we feel during the day. Mistakenly we not only attempt to heal the body with our foods but also our heart for what is overdone or missing altogether in our life.

Sugar Blues **was written by William Duffy in 1975.** He built a strong case for the addiction and psychological damage done by excess sugar consumption. I first became aware of the chemical hold of sugar on me when in Israel working on a kibbutz, a farming commune. On the day off, I traveled the countryside and ate when hungry. However, when spotting an ice cream stand I found myself ordering not one but two sundaes at a time. I had never done that before and realized how much I missed the sweet taste to which I was accustomed.

All the foods we eat have an impact on the marvelous chemistry of the body and brain. A wide array of reactions are triggered by the wonderful variety of foods from which we can choose. I'm in favor of food allergy testing to identify immune reactions. Such testing identifies the foods our immune system is attacking. These attacks spread inflammatory reactions throughout the body. The organ or organs that are affected vary according to many factors including gene predisposition.

However, how do we determine what is best for our nervous system and subsequent emotional reactions that both initiate food choices and are triggered off by them? It goes both ways. We are capable of observing our mood before we eat and the effect of the foods on our mood after we eat. We need to realize that we have a built-in testing laboratory within ourselves.

My suggestion is that we pay attention and learn from our own experiences. We are smart enough to be our own researcher for the medicine we need from the foods we choose. We can learn from the expertise and brilliance of those who study nutrition. However the foods we need for our best health depend on our own individual needs defined by what we learn about ourselves.

The psychology of eating is especially apparent in the studies that trick our senses. We can help ourselves by paying attention to research that shows that size of container matters, color of foods and container transparency all make a difference in how much food is consumed. The smaller the container, duller the color and less we see the less we eat.

Summary: 5 Steps How To Eat Well For A Healthy Long Life

Here are some steps to take and questions to ask for how to use the mind to rise above the impulses of the body and the mood:

1. **Choose the foods that are healthy:**
    a. Eat one cup of raw or cooked vegetables per meal; a variety is best; above the ground more than below the ground.

b. Lean meats or some kind of protein each meal; fish and fowl are best though lean beef and pork may work if there are no major reasons against them; powder proteins may suffice if energy levels are acceptable.
c. Consume healthy snacks in the form of nuts, dried fruit, and chewable fruits.

2. **Minimize the foods that are potentially harmful in more than modest amounts:**
   a. Minimize grains if any signs of intolerance; whole grains are healthier than white rice, bread, pasta and potatoes.
   b. Minimize or avoid sugar, salt, alcohol, coffee, juice, energy drinks and smoothies.
   c. Avoid nicotine, fried foods and sodas.
   d. Self discipline is a keynote to successfully eating! It is a skill in living that we all need to master eventually.
3. **Remember and review the best foods for the day**:
   a. Begin the day with the memories of the best of health known, whether in childhood or teens or later, enjoying the energy, alertness and independence this state of health provided during the best of times. What is a good memory of my best health ever?
   b. Review the options for breakfast, the best foods available, how healthy they will taste and how pleased the body feels after ingesting them; rehearse the morning's activities with all the energy obtained from the foods chosen; be grateful for the capacity to choose wisely and the pride with having done so.
   c. Consider the choices available for lunch; rehearse the foods digesting well, satisfied with the quality and quantity and the energy obtained for the afternoon's activities; review the events of the afternoon and possible enjoyments it may bring.
   d. Review dinner, with whom and the choices available; choose the foods most likely to be best, how well they body receives them and the energy they provide; consider healthy snacks that may be necessary later in the evening if needed; review what has gone well

through the day, the interactions in which you participated and what you added to those around you, however small; be grateful for the day, the health you have and the capacity to choose how to make it work well.

4. **Dwell on the energy, enjoyment and fulfillment you will experience this day from the foods you choose.** There are many tools of healing the body (diet, exercise, right relationships, healthy activities), healing the emotions (kindness, caring, forgiveness, tolerance, goodwill) and healing the mind (the abilities to organize, synthesize, understand, plan, aspire, learn and help others). Each of these is a nourishing food of its own energy. Look for the higher correspondences!
5. **Ask for help from the higher self.** Choose wisely the foods that will help contribute to a healthy body for the activities of the day. The old tradition of grace before meals helps to mobilize the ability to choose wisely. The purpose of optimal nutrition is to serve the purpose for living, the highest aspirations we can imagine as our life plan. This is why we need to be healthy and whole. The body serves the plan for which it was designed. This dedication in turn helps us remember how to treat the body well, lovingly, kindly and effectively.

Chapter 4

How to Revitalize with Exercise

Physical exercise springs up from the innate urge to move, to be active and interact with the world around us. It is the means whereby the body expresses its energy, enjoys life and expands its health. Exercise increases healing by ensuring the distribution of nutrients and activating the many self-lubricating joints and muscles.

Exercise is finally getting the attention it deserves. I vividly recall a medical meeting several years ago on hypertension where the national expert speaking did not even mention exercise as a treatment tool. The medical field only slowly embraced exercise as means of healing and health in the past decade and still fails to emphasize it enough. Fortunately many others in the health field are researching and teaching its mighty impact for every organ and cell of the body. Exercise is the energizing engine for excellent function of the body.

The benefits of physical exercise are immense and there are a rapidly expanding number of studies to verify it. Every organ of the body functions better with exercise: the heart, lungs, intestines, nervous system, endocrine system and even the skin.

The heart itself becomes stronger because it is pushed to work. It is a muscle, though somewhat different than the arm and leg muscles. The force of the heart beat and the need for nutrients stimulates the formation of new blood vessels. The more vessels we have the more easily blood flows to every cell, carrying oxygen, repair material and hormones. The new vessels increase the collateral circulation, which means the circulation can be adjusted quickly for rapid requirements of fresh nutrients especially in case of damage or arteriosclerosis.

A super highway system enables delivery of goods to remote areas, especially valuable in times of urgent need. More blood vessels allow for routing through difficult regions of compromised tissue. Such service becomes increasingly important as the body ages and hardening of the arteries diminishes blood flow. In case of a major vessel obstruction as in a heart attack or stroke, a rich collateral circulation can compensate quickly and minimize the damage.

The lungs transfer oxygen from the air into the blood stream. Oxygen is the single most important element without which we cannot survive. Exercise increases the blood flow to and through the lungs. The more numerous the vessels the more efficiently the oxygen is absorbed. Exercise also increases the number of red blood cells produced by the bone marrow which means there are more oxygen-carrying vehicles available.

The other main function of the lungs is to discharge carbon dioxide. This is a common waste product of metabolism; its elimination is necessary for optimal oxygen saturation. In emphysema lung tissue is slowly destroyed, decreasing the carbon dioxide discharge and oxygen-carrying capacity. In bronchitis and asthma the flow of air is compromised by inflamed, swollen tissues and restricted bronchioles that limit air exchange. Exercise expands the number of blood vessels in the lungs that enables the production of a higher number of breathing tubules, allowing better function especially in the presence of disease.

Exercise outside and in nature also has added benefits. The sun is a powerful force of energy besides the warmth and light. Of course the warmth increases the circulation to the surface of the body, including the nose, throat and sinuses for immune protective functions. This is one of the reasons that colds and the flu are more common in the winter months. We are not only in closed spaces with sick people but our immune screening systems rely on optimal circulation in the mouth, nose and throat areas. In cooler weather these areas decrease the blood supply to preserve energy.

The intestines perform multiple complex functions of digestion, assimilation and elimination. Healthy blood flow from exercise maximizes stomach function so that sufficient acid and protective buffering mucus is available for turning the food into a pudding-like consistency. The pancreas is even more complex with its double function of secreting digestive enzymes and also as an endocrine organ. The digestive enzymes are produced for the three major food groups of carbohydrates, fats and proteins. The endocrine function of the pancreas is its secretion of insulin, which decreases sugar in the blood and the counter-balancing hormone, glucagon, which increases it. As we age exercise is essential to optimize these functions.

After eating more than a modest meal there is a common tendency to feel slightly more sluggish. This occurs as a result of shunting some of the blood flow from the brain to supply the increased circulation to the abdomen for its digestive functions. There is also decreased circulation to the muscles, which is why we are strongly advised not to swim after eating. Swimming increases the need for nutrients while digestion diminishes the capacity to deliver them. This results in mineral depletion, muscle cramping and possible immobility in the water. Exercise diminishes these tendencies for blood flow limits.

Exercise enhances blood flow to the intestines enabling optimal acid secretion from the stomach and enzyme production from the pancreas ensuring better breakdown of food substances. Less than a full flow of enzymes leads to partially digested food particles in the blood stream that contributes to the development of food allergy and sensitivity. Immune reactions to these larger than healthy-sized substances lead to a variety of systemic conditions including fatigue, headaches and skin problems. Lack of good digestive ability allows more nutrients to end up in the large intestine where they become food for billions of bacteria. The byproduct is gas leading to bloating and other congestive symptoms. Exercise helps prevent these problems.

The nervous system requires good blood flow to deliver basic nutrients for new cell growth and energizing activity. Contrary to old science the nervous system is continuously regenerating itself though at a slower pace than the other organs. There is growing recognition that nerve hormone function depends on basic protein delivery. Optimal blood flow from exercise helps to ensure high nerve hormone levels which sustain the abilities to focus, understand, remember and follow through with plans for the day. Also largely unrecognized is the nervous system as a major source of energy. It requires optimal exercise for full function capacity.

The endocrine system is a major communicator of changes within the body and the environment. Hormones are complex chemicals that have functions distant from where they are secreted. They are like ambassadors to every organ of the body, and also require the right amount of nutrient flow through the blood stream for healthy function. All hormone function begins to diminish as we age for many reasons, one of which is insufficient exercise. Unless the nutrient delivery continues at a full pace, aging accelerates faster than necessary.

The most intriguing aspect of the hormone system is that every cell has receptor entry points for every major hormone. There are built-in doorways for every hormone. But unless delivered in good amounts to each cell through optimal blood flow, the doorways will be undeveloped and underutilized. The hormones are the greatest source of cell energy and regeneration. Exercise is essential to ensure their full use. Hormone secretion is also stimulated by the sun, the exposure to which is more likely with a good exercise routine outdoors.

Even the skin relies on exercise to be healthy. Exercise is probably the main reason we are outside in the air. Exposure to the sun is the best way to stimulate the production of vitamin D, now considered a hormone. It affects every organ of the body with evidence showing its capacity to minimize blood sugar, cholesterol and cancer risk. One of the reasons for decreased health, energy and mood in the winter months is the decreased exposure to the sun. Although we can take supplements of vitamin D, it must still reach every cell to provide its benefits to them. This is done in large part by the pumping action of the heart that requires a good exercise effort.

One of the reasons for aging skin and risk for skin cancer is insufficient delivery of the immune cells to the skin. Areas of decreased circulation limit the nutrient supply and allow for bruising and slower repair of damaged tissues. The skin is an elimination organ, responsible for 5% of body waste removal. Optimal circulation from good exercise helps the skin fulfill this mission of detoxification, ensuring greater vitality and longer youthful appearance.

What types of exercise should I do?

There are three major types of exercise: stretching, cardiovascular and weight lifting. There are many ways to do each of these. Personal benefit depends on individual needs, preferences and willingness to perform exercise in a consistent manner.

Stretching exercises have a long history of use but only a recent need. As we have evolved to a very sedentary way of living stretching time has become more necessary. The oldest well-known form of exercise is Yoga, especially Hatha Yoga. There are many forms of Yoga for the heart, mind and spirit, but Hatha is mainly used for the physical conditioning. Tai Chi is probably just as old though not quite as popular. Pilates is a relative newcomer exercise of growing interest, well adapted for the modern health minded.

Over the years I've seen many forms spring up, become popular and then diminish. The popularity of a particular type usually stems more from the charisma of the originator than anything else. The best form of stretching exercise is the one you do regularly. If you have special physical conditions of concern, private instruction may be necessary. Physical therapists are trained to do exercise training for medical musculoskeletal problems. A growing number of personal trainers are also supplying this need for individual instruction.

The benefit of stretching is to lubricate the major joints and tone up the major muscle groups. Cardiovascular conditioning is not enough as the body ages to adequately ensure joint flexibility. Most cardio exercise is repetitive without full range of motion of major muscles and joints. Often older folks comment on popping, crackling and other sounds when beginning to stretch. These diminish and usually disappear with a daily routine. Anyone with chronic neck or back pain should stretch twice daily while the conditions continue. Janet Travel, M.D. did research at Cornell Medical Center 50 years ago showing that 70% of musculoskeletal pain conditions that did not involve nerve damage recover with a regular stretching program.

I often recommend a daily dozen set of stretches. Most people need some form of daily stretching when reaching age 40, although anyone with neck or back pain conditions will need them earlier. It is usually best to start slowly, increasing the number of repetitions as able and needed.

Cardiovascular exercise is a modern requirement to extend health and healing. It was first popularized by Dr. Ken Cooper in the 1970s. His first book is *The Aerobics Way.* In it he describes the oxygen-enhancing effect with vigorous exercise. He reviewed research and conducted numerous studies showing that elevating the heart rate for designated periods of time improved the health of every organ, especially the heart and blood vessel system. There is definite decreased disease incidence and increased recovery rate for many conditions with optimal aerobic exercise.

Dr. Cooper carefully measured the effects of intense exercise. He established guidelines for how much exercise needs to be done to meet a minimal requirement for cardiovascular fitness for a wide range of exercises. For example, optimal aerobic walking requires covering three miles in 45 minutes on a daily basis. I usually recommend a slower pace for one hour. More vigorous exercise like biking, swimming or jogging require only 20-30 minutes for the same effect as long as moderate exertion is applied. The shortest time exercise that meets this level requirement is jogging in place; it only takes 12.5 minutes but requires lifting the feet at least 4 inches with each step and taking 2 steps/second.

There is growing research in the area of interval training. This requires fast to maximum exertion for 1-2 minute periods followed by 1-2 minute slow periods repeated 5-7 times as a daily routine. The research is compelling on the benefits achieved for the heart, hypertension, hyperlipidemia, weight reduction and vitality.

Lifting weights is very beneficial for strengthening major muscle groups. It is definitely therapeutic for a wide range of musculoskeletal conditions and essential for some. This is the type of exercise most likely to require expert advice unless you have prior experience and know how to start slowly and carefully. The size of muscle is not as important as tone and basic strength for common activities. Weight lifting increases muscle mass and decreases fat mass. Many feel best when lifting weights regularly.

No matter the age one starts muscles can be strengthened to some degree. Studies show that men in their 70s can begin weight training that significantly increases carrying capacity, repetitive lifting time and recovery from injury. Exercise also increases self care and independence for a longer time.

A few comments about osteoporosis are worth making. Weight bearing exercise such as walking, jogging and jumping has been promoted as the healthiest way to increase bone mass. Further research now shows that every kind of exercise increases bone mass, though weight bearing is still the most able to do so. However, exercise also increases agility, flexibility and reflex reaction. These may even be more important than bone density as they increase our capacity for preventing falls from weakness or awkwardness.

Adverse Effects Of Exercise

The most common adverse effects of exercise is not doing it and suffering from the lack of exercise. Problems can occur but do not come close to the poor health likely to result from not doing enough. Just as every organ system improves with exercise, every organ suffers from an insufficient amount.

Stretching exercises cause problems with over-stretching. I see patients who over-stretch creating a new strain that can last several weeks, even months. This also occurs in guided group classes. The most common cause is lack of attention to what the body can handle. This is especially likely over the age of 40 and when re-starting a routine after not exercising for several months or years. There is an assumption that we can do what we always used to be able to do. However, as the body ages, it also contracts. The tissues lose flexibility and range of motion. It takes more time to reach a high level of fitness as we age than when younger. The risk for over-stretching is diminished by taking more time, especially when beginning a new regimen. At times a personal trainer will over-coach, especially with an older client. Everyone can stretch at least a little. At the Pain Clinic everyone could do the exercises at least to some degree and were much better for doing it. Everyone increased their capacity as they performed it daily. If those with chronic pain can exercise daily so can the rest of us.

Cardiovascular exercise is more likely to cause a wide range of problems. With cardio exercise adverse effects may not be known until the next day or two. Unexpected fatigue, neck or back pain may occur. More serious problems could affect the heart, though this is rare. Chest pain, pressure or shortness of breath soon after exercising are possible signs of insufficient circulation to the heart and should lead to medical assessment. There has been some concern that advanced athletes incur an enlarged heart from excess exercise with the assumption that the heart is weaker as a result. Further studies indicate that heavy exercisers with larger hearts have healthier ones, too. Some vigorous exercisers also refer to their routine as addictive. My observation is that when people miss the exercise for a period of time they miss the vitality they gain from it. This is a positive addiction with some exceptions such as anorexia, underweight and loss of menstrual function due to exercise.

Weight training leads to sore muscles, but it is part of the training effect. If the pain continues to worsen, it may be necessary to stop for a few days and lighten the routine. Serious disease from weight training is uncommon, though I know one man who fractured his arm by over-lifting. The ideal role of the mind in exercising is to cooperate with the needs and limits of the body, not impose unrealistic expectations. Any new or worsening pain condition from exercise should be given medical attention.

How Much Is Enough?

The amount of exercise needed depends on the goals. An ideal program for most will include stretching 10-15 minutes per day. Stretching is recommended before vigorous cardio to prevent over stretching and over use of the muscles used. As the body ages, cardio is not enough to ensure full range of motion of major joints and muscles. As muscles age or become strained adjustments may be necessary. It is often helpful to consider new ways of improving the routine to make it more interesting, effective and enjoyable.

When should stretching exercises be done? I have heard people warned about stretching in the morning because the body is stiffer, especially as it ages. I think this is a good reason to stretch first thing in the morning. It helps wake up the body and get it ready for the day. But this is a personal issue. The most important time to stretch is when it works best for your typical day.

Cardiovascular exercise should meet optimal aerobic needs of the body. The Aerobics guidelines include distances, times and amount of work done in calculating the amount needed for excellent heart and blood vessel activity. Walking one hour per day at a moderate rate is a very healthy goal. More vigorous exercise like jogging, biking or swimming takes less time, usually 30 minutes per day. Those who prefer more vigorous workouts may establish a 3-5 day per week routine instead of a daily one.

When cardio exercise should be done depends on the schedule that works best. I like to exercise first thing in the morning but others prefer the noontime and some after a day's work. The timing is not as important as the doing of it.

The amount of weight training depends on the goal. If the goal is building specific muscle groups to increase strength for daily activities, then 2-3 times/week works well. If the goal is building a prominent muscle for appearance or performance, much more work and effort are required. For such a goal it is usually a good idea to work with an individual trainer, at least initially.

What Is The Role Of Exercise On Emotional Well-being?

Exercise for emotional well-being has several factors to it. Primarily exercise increases our contact with other people and that is the main reason for its positive emotional impact. However, there are physical components to exercise that add to our sense of well-being. Many studies confirm the value of exercise in decreasing anxiety, depression and other psychic states of dysfunction.

Physically, exercise increases the nutrients and subsequent functioning of every organ of the body. There is a greater sense of vitality that increases the hormone supply and the nervous system in particular. These add to the general amount of energy and responsiveness to interact with those around us. Physical exercise gives a sense of physical confidence in how the body feels and appears that also increases our sense of who we are and willingness to share it with others.

The light of the sun stimulates the hormones systems of the body. Vitamin D is the main chemical stimulated by the light of the sun. Its functions include aiding the immune system. Although initial studies do not support an infection protection function, there is intriguing evidence that we have much more to learn about how it helps us. It benefits the function of every organ of the body. In addition to increasing D levels, all the other hormone systems are increased with exposure to the sun. This means that the energy hormones of the thyroid, adrenal and gender gland hormones are increased as well. Increased energy increases our interest in interacting with others and the life around us that in turn increases our general sense of well-being and healing energy streaming through our body.

Exercise can increase our contact with others. Interactions with others are the real key to greater expressiveness, confidence and enjoyment of living. The more people around us, the more likely we will hear how others are doing and share who we are. It is the activity of interaction that stimulates the feeling state. When we express what we feel we get a better sense of what there is inside us and other's response to us.

Exercise can increase our exposure to nature and its many life forms. Flowers, bushes, and trees add beauty and joyfulness if we take the time to notice and interact with intention. Streams, rivers and lakes often provide a calming, quieting influence. Elevated views of the surrounding area give us perspective and an opportunity to rise above the usual routines. Mountain views inspire aspiration and hope for something better. Sunrises, sunsets and the night sky can elevate us to grander views of what is possible and the larger scheme of life of which we are a part, and inspirations from which we can draw. All of which boosts the mood and mind and becomes more available with outdoor exercise.

Extreme Exercise

Extreme exercise is for something other than physical health. It is important to realize and accept this. There may be many reasons to do so that may be very valid and worthwhile. There are stories of people given a poor prognosis who pour huge amounts of energy into major physical exertion. In the process they also energize the immune system and major healing occurs. The healing is a result of the new conviction to turn their life into a productive one. The miles run or the mountain climbed is not the source of the healing as much as the new optimism and determination to make life worthwhile.

Beyond physical fitness, what is the reason for extreme exercise? My favorite insight from Dr. Cooper is his statement about the four types of exercisers. He says that there are beginners, intermediates and advanced athletes. However, the fourth type is the most important, the mature exerciser. That is the one who only does enough to be healthy. More exercise than is needed for health is for reasons other than health of body. At times people pursue exercise to compensate for what is missing in life, in terms of confidence or sense of well being. It is worthwhile to be honest about the goals and expectations.

The sad part of extreme exercise is that it increases the risk for infection, injury and disease. Many high exercisers become ill after the long race or cycle ride and require several days to recover. There are ways to prevent these reactions with optimal nutrition, supplements and conditioning. However, it is still important to answer the question of the need for doing it. Unfortunately some individuals suffer loss of limb and life in pursuing intense activities.

Extreme exercise is for something other than physical health. It is important to realize and accept this clearly. At times people pursue an intense physical exercise routine assuming it is the most important way to ensure health. When they come down with an illness they are surprised the physical exertion didn't protect them. Consulting with our inner being and the larger plan and purpose of our life can help minimize such risks and help maintain a healthy perspective. In the process we may learn to what extent we are dependent upon physical stimulation for filling our life with meaningful experience. There is much more to our health than a healthy body. We also need a healthy heart, mind and spirit. The best exercise may be bending over to help someone else with their life.

The Ultimate Purpose of Exercise

The main reason to exercise is to have a healthy body for the purpose of expressing the heart, mind and soul. These need a vehicle of expression that can be relied upon. It is similar to the value of having a new computer compared to an old one. The new one works faster, with more functions, fewer problems and greater ease. A new computer doesn't guarantee quality of use, content of messages or use of important information available. It enables better expression of feeling, thinking and meaningful activity.

A healthy body enables us to use the five senses in enlightened ways if we are creative in our efforts. It provides the energy we need to put in a full day's work. A healthy body helps us interact with others in a dependable, understandable way. It helps us communicate more reliably for a longer period of time with those around us with the intelligence and emotions that we have developed.

An unhealthy body inhibits our ability to have the stamina it needs for a full day. If it is easily fatigued or achy our tolerance for physical and emotional activity is diminished, at times severely. An unhealthy body lacks the ability to accurately sense what we see and hear, compromising communication with those with whom we associate. It is less able to access memories and connect them to make sense of our daily events and interactions.

The highest aspects of our heart, mind and spirit cherish a healthy body to fulfill their missions. It can do so without a totally healthy body and does so in many people. However, to express our caring, compassion and cheerfulness it helps to have a healthy body. To express our alertness, awareness, focus, skills and talents that add life to our family, friends and community, it helps to have a healthy body. A healthy body is one that serves the higher function of our innate capacities, instead of just experiencing the world of sensation. The ultimate function of the body is to contribute to the well being of those around us to the best of our abilities and be gracious to those who help make our life livable and enjoyable.

Chapter 5

Serene Sleep Strategies

Sleep is the time for rest and renewal of the body. All the organs are cleansed and nourished during the hours of sleep. The immune maintenance crew wakes up and goes to work at night, healing and renewing us. Almost all my patients who are well and enjoying their life have a good night's rest. They awaken refreshed and look forward to the day. Those with insomnia disorders are tired, weaker and more likely to be moody. Fortunately there are many strategies for successful sleep.

It is now recognized that there are five stages of sleep. The nighttime state of sleep is a bit more complicated than most realize. Since the early extensive studies at sleep clinics in the 1950s, a great deal of investigation has explored the dark hours of sleep. Sleep scientists define them by electroencephalogram (EEG) and clinical changes. The clinical changes are easier to understand.

* Stage 1 is early, light sleep, easily awakened, associated with mild muscle twitching. The heart and breathing rate begin to lessen. This stage lasts 10-20 minutes.
* Stage 2 is a deeper version, less easily awakened, with unlikely muscle action and lasting 10-20 minutes.
* Stage 3 is early deep sleep when muscle activity is suppressed, and the circulation is increased to the intestines for digestion, assimilation and elimination; it lasts 10-20 minutes.

* Stage 4 is deep sleep, when most of the renewal and regeneration occurs. During this stage heart and breathing rate are at their lowest levels. Cell debris is most efficiently removed and nutrients are delivered more fully to each individual cell.
* Stage 5 is rapid eye movement sleep, called REM sleep. This is dream time. When we are awakened during stages 1-4, dream activity is reported only 6% of the time. When awakened during REM sleep, dreams are identified 86% of the time. The dreams of non-REM time are passive, slow and generally uninteresting. REM sleep dreams are usually quite active, with mixtures of recognizable, reasonable events and people along with quite bizarre, unusual activity.

During the night we have 3-4 Stage 4 periods, decreasing in length from an initial 30-40 minutes to 5-10 minutes. The REM times progressively lengthen from an initial 10-15 minutes up to 30-40 minutes. As we age, sleep length decreases from early childhood of 12-14 hours to 6-8 hours/night. There is also decreasing stage 4 and REM sleep, although both continue and are necessary for optimal health.

Healthy sleep is one of the three most basic elements of physical health and well being, along with optimal nutrition and exercise. We are designed to spend a quarter to a third of our lives sleeping. Without enough we quickly become irritable, sluggish, fatigued and intolerant of minor stressors. We are at increased risk for many illnesses. Most diseases are made worse by insufficient sleep, especially pain, fatigue and memory loss. Even weight gain, infections and cancer are being associated with inadequate sleep time. Insufficient sleep is the second most common cause of car accidents. It is the cause of several prominent tragedies including the Three Mile Island radiation leak, the Bhopal (India) nuclear accident and the Challenger Space Shuttle accident. These were all related to personnel or supervisory staff without adequate sleep and subsequent dysfunctional reaction time misjudgments.

We all need enough sleep. How much is enough? It varies to a certain degree, but most adults need 7-9 hours/night. More important is the quality of sleep rather than the amount. Many of my patients who complain of fatigue and tiredness have fitful sleep. Some get enough sleep or even more than average and still awaken tired. This is a sign of metabolic abnormalities, often nutritional and hormonal as well as unresolved accumulated stress.

Causes of insufficient and low quality sleep vary widely. The obvious question to ask is when the problem began and what events occurred within a few days to weeks prior to the onset of trouble. Starting a new medication is usually easy to catch. Sleep can also be affected by new supplements, vitamins, herbs or hormones. Less obvious to many is a change of diet. Especially as we age, the capacity for digesting and assimilating certain foods lessens. More complicated foods may well congest the system when they did not do so at a younger age. Alcohol, soda, spices, chocolate and caffeine may contribute to poor sleep.

Many illnesses can interfere with sleep. New onset of a pain condition or worsening of a chronic pain condition such as headaches or migraines will often interfere with sleep. Irritable bowel syndrome, fibromyalgia, nasal congestion, chest congestion, allergies, asthma and many other conditions will interfere with sleep. And, of course, inadequate sleep will worsen most medical conditions.

The most common cause of sleep disruption is emotional, our reaction to stressful events. Work issues or worries of serious illness in yourself, spouse, family or close friend often is the source of stress. Disagreement with anyone we are close to or work with may be a problem, especially if it goes unresolved for more than a few days. Frustration or anger with those we do not know is usually a sign of low tolerance, inflexibility or lack of priorities. A tendency for pessimism or depression predisposes vulnerability to common stressors.

The real cause of emotional distress is a lack of the ability to respond to life's challenges with creativity. Often the initial reaction to troublesome news is an emotional one. As we apply thoughtfulness and willingness to explore causal connections we can consider more options for action. As we apply calmness, we can gain time for reflection and other's views. As we seek broader meaning we can see the trigger of an event as one piece of a larger puzzle and better activate the need to restrain ourselves more effectively for long-term goals.

Sometimes the loss of sleep is due to a greater service we seek to provide like having a new child. Babies require huge amounts of attention and time, especially at night. But we give it willingly, at least at first, because we love the life within the child and want to do all we can to nurture his/her needs whenever they arise.

I have a patient with such a special project. She and her husband have a major film project for children. Started by her husband's father, they brought it back to life and found an eager audience to watch it. However the work to bring it to life is very consuming requiring much traveling and interacting with a variety of people, some of whom are very difficult and have their own idea how the film should unfold. She is struggling with a sleep problem made worse by playing a major role in this project. Because she knows the value of it she is willing to sacrifice herself and sleep to do it right and do it well. This is a healthy sleep problem. As she gains insight in how to master the art of the work while including recognition of her own needs, she grows, learns and accomplishes the challenges before her.

The treatment of insomnia has many options including medications, supplements, herbs, and mental housecleaning. There are many common medications that enhance sleep and many others that are used off-label (i.e. officially for another neurological problem) but very effective for sleep as well, such as estrogen and progesterone. Many alternative treatments work as well including supplements used in the therapeutic range.

Sleep Treatment Suggestions

1. **Melatonin** is a natural nerve hormone the body secretes to induce sleep. As a supplement it is safe, sometimes effective and has multiple benefits (energy, immune stimulation, anti-aging). The optimal dose varies from 0.5-10mg. Adverse effects are uncommon but occur in the form of sluggish awakening and restless sleep. Doses beyond 3mg

should be in collaboration with a physician. As with most supplements if there is trouble getting to sleep it is best to take one hour before desired sleep time. If the problem is awaking early then doses may be taken at bedtime.

2. **Kava Kava** is a South Pacific herb that is sedating. It may help to induce and maintain sleep. A small number of serious liver problems have occurred in those taking massive amounts. If you have liver enzyme elevations do not use this one. 2-3 capsules at bedtime is usually sufficient.
3. **Magnesium citrate** is the most absorbable form of magnesium. This is a common mineral that relaxes muscle and nerve action. It is safe, inexpensive and potentially helpful. If too much is taken, diarrhea may occur. 250-500mg is a good dose.
4. **Sleep supplement combination remedies**. Most of these have herbs that are helpful but usually present only in modest amounts. They are worth trying and usually free of adverse effects.
5. **Medications** for insomnia disorders. At times medications work only for limited periods of time. When that is the case I recommend rotating two or more in a cyclic fashion to make the most of them.
6. **Optimal exercise** is the key to some people's aid to sleep. Exercise flushes out debris from cell activity allowing muscles and nerves to move into a relaxed state throughout the night. Significant exertion may be required to induce sleep, however, not within an hour or so before bedtime.
7. **Learning how to shift from the awake active state to the relaxed state** of the nervous system at bedtime is very important. We are born problem solvers and many overdo by obsessing about worries, concerns, duties and deadlines when they go to bed. The way to shift from the problem solving brain to the relaxing brain is to review the best events of the day in the early evening; i.e. what went well, what you enjoyed, compliments received or gratitude extended to others. Savor the best one as you go to sleep.

8. **Relaxation exercises** have been available for millennia. These are still not learned or used enough for most people with sleep disorders. Training and daily practice will benefit those who make the effort. Some CDs are exceptional such as those by Norm Shealy and Belleruth Naparstek.

Relaxing Exercises

Relaxation is mainly a mental exercise that trains the body to focus on images and suggestions that shift the nervous system to a soothing, serene state.

The simplest relaxing exercise is to recall a memory of being relaxed. It can be anywhere anytime. For some the best memory is being in bed and not having to work the next day. For others it may be at the end of the day, able to relax and visit with family or friends. A relaxing memory may be a favorite vacation, a beautiful landscape view, a mountain view or being on the beach in a warm summer day. The memory is like a web site that can recreate the sensations of relaxing just by dwelling on it and enjoying it.

A simple relaxing exercise at bedtime is to follow these steps to induce relaxing sleep:

1. Close the eyes, take in a deep breath and invite the body into a relaxed state. The body enjoys relaxing especially after a full day's activity.
2. Start at the head sensing how it feels, asking it to let go and to relax. Be aware of the forehead. If there is any sensation of tightness, ask that to stop. "Forehead, relax." Repeat three times.
3. Appreciate whatever response occurs and invite that to flow downwards across the eyes. If there is any tightness or strain in the eyes, ask that to stop. "Eyes relax."
4. Proceed to each body part, the jaws, neck, shoulders, arms, hands, chest, abdomen, back, legs, feet and toes. Each in turn is felt, registered and asked to relax, to be comfortable then to flow downwards to the next part.
5. You can also start at the feet and work your way upwards with similar suggestions.

There is also the Jacobsen Relaxation Technique. This was developed by an American physician, Edmund Jacobson, in the early 1920s. It involves tightening then relaxing each muscle group, one by one, until the whole body is involved. The starting point is usually the right hand, tightening then relaxing 1-3 times. Each time the part is tightened it is helpful to study how it feels and watch how tension spreads. Then move to the forearm, the upper arm, the shoulder and the neck. Move to the other side of the body in the same fashion. Each muscle is connected to another like the old song says. With each muscle contraction and relaxation there is a refractory period where the muscle cannot tighten near as readily and thus naturally feels more relaxed. It takes more energy than some want to exert at night and some in fact become more awake with this exercise. However many do respond.

There are many relaxing exercises on the Internet. The goal is to find one that works consistently and then use it regularly. Some may have to experiment with relaxing during the day to develop the skill so that it works at night. Others can only practice at night when tired.

Mental Housecleaning Induces Sleep

At times relaxing is not enough. The body responds but the emotions and mind remain awake and alert. Then the need is to develop a way to unwind the events of the day. We have to put things in order, assess the events and emotions of the day and process them.

Mental housecleaning is the process of surveying what happened during the day and put it to rest. The most worrisome events and feelings are usually the ones that come to mind first. Each should be dealt with on its own. Review what happened, what was learned, and possible reasonable steps that can be taken tomorrow that will address the concern. Use the imagination to create how you would like it to go.

Accept the strengths that became noticeable or consider the strengths needed to make it acceptable. If anxiety is present ask for calmness or reassurance of a good decision made. If fear is present ask for confidence or conviction of a cherished truth. If doubt about what to do occurs ask for advice from a wise, trusted friend or mentor about what to do. If guilt is present ask for forgiveness and accept the lesson learned that will be easier to express next time such an event happens. A contented heart and mind enables sleep more than most medications!

The Joys of Insomnia

When I worked with Dr. Loomis at the Meadowlark Retreat Center, he noticed that as he aged he began to have sleep changes. But it didn't take him long to turn it around. When asked about sleep from the Center's guests he would often launch into a wonderful talk about the joys of insomnia. He would see the middle of the night as an excellent time to review the love received from others, the love given to family, friends and guests, successes and proud moments. He would use this time to review peak events that celebrate life. At times he would commune with the source of life itself. For him this was usually an experience in nature, like blazing a new walking trail on his property. Enjoyable events are worth celebrating over and over and can enrich an evening without sleep as well. The middle of the night is a quiet time when there is little distraction of business, noises and common sounds. It allows more clear thinking time and a chance to request help from the deep well of our inner being. Evarts learned how to use it well and so can each of us.

Chapter 6

How to Find the Harmony of Hormone Balance

The hormone system is an extraordinary complex of dynamic energy centers. Hormones are complex chemicals designed to function in harmony like a wonderful symphony of many sounds. The hormone glands have multiple ways of vitalizing, maintaining and regenerating every organ and cell of the body. The hormone system has recently become an area of high interest in integrative medicine because of its impact in treating and preventing chronic disease and the entire aging process.

What is a hormone and how do they work? A hormone is a complex chemical secreted by a hormone gland that has an effect on every cell of the body. It is derived from a Greek word meaning impetus or impulse that is the energy or force to set in motion. When hormones are surging energy is rising. Most treatment for hormone dysfunction refers to deficiency states and how to replenish them. The use of estrogen and progesterone are probably most well-known but there are many other critical hormones.

Hormones are primarily messengers of cell activity and interaction with the environment. They are the means whereby the body communicates with itself, adjusts itself and prepares for upcoming activities. They are an integral part of an elaborate internal communication system.

The effects of hormones are vast. They include vitality, sexual drive, reproduction, cell metabolism, bone growth, muscle strength, intestinal function, appetite change, immune system function, alertness, memory and more. Virtually every cell of the body is affected by a wide range of hormones, and thus every function of the body requires multiple hormone involvement.

The major hormone glands are called endocrine because they secrete hormones directly into the blood stream. Most organs of the body have a local effect in the region of the body where they reside. In other words, the muscle of the forearm moves the arm so you can scratch your nose. The kidneys clean the blood stream as it flows through them. But hormone secretions affect organs and cells in all parts of the body.

Hormones work like a key in a lock. To enter a cell the hormone must find the lock it fits into, the receptor molecule. Various factors determine the level of hormone secreted, the number of receptor sites available and how well they interact with one another. All of these are influenced by our genetic tendencies, foods, fluids, feelings and relationships.

The hormones I will discuss are thyroid, adrenal, gender (estrogen, progesterone, testosterone), intestinal and neurotransmitter nerve hormones. Each one is described in terms of its functions, symptoms of dysfunction, methods to measure, ways to treat and adverse effects. The final section addresses the lifestyle effects as causes of hormone dysfunction and as a means to optimize their function.

Thyroid Hormones

Thyroid dysfunction is recognized as a common endocrine disorder often seen by primary care doctors. Hypothyroidism (insufficient amounts of the hormone) is the most common thyroid problem. It is estimated to affect 5-20% of the population, depending on how you define it. Generally 10% of women have hypothyroidism by age 50 and close to 20% by age 60. I suspect it is even higher.

Over 100 years ago, it was medically recorded and recognized that many people suffered from goiter, an enlarged thyroid gland. Enlargement occurs as a result of iodine deficiency. The gland compensates by making more hormone-producing cells. Some goiters became so large that people had so much trouble breathing and swallowing that surgery was performed on many of them. As a result of surgery and loss of the thyroid gland we learned about significant problems associated with thyroid deficiency.

In 1888, a British Commission studied 100 patients with severe hypothyroidism, especially affecting menstrual function and energy level. In 1891, thyroid therapy became available and many problems from thyroid deficiency became reversible.

Early therapy was prepared from animal thyroid extracts (beef, pork and lamb), the first being injectable sheep thyroid. Dried thyroid tablets became available soon thereafter. Potency varies a bit depending on the health of the animal. At times, the tri-iodo thyronine, T3, portion became excessive because it is produced in higher amounts in animals than humans.

Tetra-iodo thyronine, T4, thyroid was synthesized in 1950, and is the current common form of treatment because it is considered slightly more reliable. It is bio-identical, exactly as the body makes it, even though all forms are synthetic. However, many physicians prefer the more complete animal thyroid medication because it has the whole range of thyroid hormones in it, T1-T4.

Thyroid hormones are major sources of energy and vitality. The purpose of thyroid hormones is to enhance oxygen use inside the cell, which affects metabolism, energy level and body heat. It also aids regulation of tissue growth, nervous and reproductive system development. Thyroid hormones modulate protein, fat and carbohydrate metabolism. They regulate vitamin use and assist in digestion.

By increasing cell activity thyroid hormones speed up many organ functions like the heart rate, blood flow and heat in the body carried by the circulating blood flow. They also increase HDL cholesterol, the good type. Thyroid hormones decrease other risk factors for heart disease like blood pressure, C-reactive protein (CRP, an inflammation marker) and homocysteine (a protein used in metabolism). Thyroid decreases the bad cholesterol, LDL, and the diastolic blood pressure (the 2nd number when the BP is taken).

Thyroid hormones increase intestinal activity allowing food and residue to be processed and eliminated efficiently. It stimulates the immune system and thus plays a role in preventing infection and cancer. They increase brain alertness, concentration and memory.

Causes of low thyroid function are most often due to aging. Family history plays a role. I also see stress as a trigger. Initially thyroid dysfunction begins as an increase in thyroid hormone production to meet increasing demands of life. Over a period of time there is a wearing out of thyroid production and diminished levels of secretion occur. Often hypothyroidism occurs after having Hashimoto's Thyroiditis, an autoimmune disorder detected by immune antibodies in the blood. The body's immune system sees the thyroid gland as foreign to the body.

Women are more likely to have low thyroid function than men, and the levels commonly begin to decline in the peri-menopausal (before menopause starts) time. I routinely begin thyroid testing in all women and most men in their 40s and find that many feel and function better with thyroid treatment.

Common symptoms of low thyroid function are a result of decreased energy affecting every organ of the body. The most obvious symptoms are fatigue, coldness and constipation. There is usually an increased weight gain, cold hands and feet and increased cholesterol levels. There may be morning stiffness, fluid retention, dry skin and brittle hair. Mental symptoms may include depression, slow thinking, decreased memory and poor concentration.

Blood tests are the most common and convenient way to measure thyroid levels. Most labs will do free T4, free T3, TSH, reverse T3 and thyroid antibodies. As the thyroid function decreases there is an increase in TSH (Thyroid Stimulating Hormone) and decrease in T3 and T4. The medical community favors TSH levels between 0.5-4.5. But there is growing interest based on studies of patient assessments that the optimal TSH should be less than 3.0. In addition to lower TSH levels, I look for upper half of normal levels of T3 and T4 for optimal function. The reverse T3 is a nonfunctioning form of T3 and should therefore be lower for best function of the gland.

In 2003 the American Association of Clinical Endocrinologists released a statement saying that TSH values over 3.0 may indicate evolving hypothyroidism. They also said that some members begin thyroid treatment above 2.0. The National Academy of Clinical Biochemistry did a thorough review of studies on thyroid function. They state that 95% of normal thyroid individuals have a TSH between 0.5 and 2.5.

Ultra sound imaging tests may be indicated when there is any abnormality of the thyroid gland, especially when there are nodules or general enlargement.

Thyroid treatment is primarily prescription thyroid. While most of the medical community favors a synthetic form of T4, a growing number favor animal thyroid that includes T4 and T3. Studies support more favorable responses to thyroid treatment when the whole thyroid gland is used. The response is improved when medication is taken upon awaking and before food. We usually start with modest amounts and increase the dose slowly as needed.

Nutritional supplements that are necessary for healthy thyroid function include iodine, selenium, zinc and tyrosine. Iodine used to be readily available in table salt but now is present only 20% of the time. Selenium helps the immune system from autoimmune reactivity. Tyrosine is the amino acid building block for thyroid hormone; some need this for optimal function. Coffee, soy and fruit juices inhibit thyroid absorption as do the supplements calcium and chromium. This is the reason thyroid medication is recommended to be taken upon arising and ideally one hour before breakfast. However, for best compliance it may still be more convenient and sufficiently effective if taken with breakfast.

Adverse effects from thyroid medication occur infrequently. These can be minimized by starting with a low dose with gradual increments as needed. Adverse effects are from over-stimulation of organ function. Over-stimulation of the heart leads to increased or irregular heart rate and possibly atrial fibrillation. Over-stimulation of the intestines to diarrhea and of the nervous system to anxiety and insomnia. If overdone for lengthy periods of time bone density may diminish as well. Follow-up testing and clinical assessment is recommended for best results.

The healing benefits of thyroid treatment are common and at times dramatic. I saw a middle-aged male recently who had been more tired, colder and with less stamina than his friends since early high school. He had irregular bowel habits and frequently dry skin and lips. Upon reaching therapeutic doses of thyroid medication he felt better than at any time in his life, after more than 20 years as an adult. Quality of life is commonly improved with optimal thyroid activity.

Adrenal Hormones

The adrenal glands are probably the first hormone glands to under-function as we age. I learned about its practical value when working with Dr. Loomis at Meadowlark. He was using adrenal cortex extract (ACE) injections for patients with fatigue and low stamina, and it was very effective for many. ACE was an injectable form of whole adrenal gland extracted from beef adrenal glands. Unfortunately the FDA banned it in the early 1980s, possibly to allow a pharmaceutical company to use the acronym in promoting a new class of anti-hypertensive medication called angiotensin converting enzyme inhibitor, ACE inhibitors for short. Over the counter adrenal tablets are widely available and used by many.

The adrenal glands sit on top of the kidneys. They are small pyramid-shaped tissues that weigh only about an ounce each, but they secrete about 150 hormones. The primary function is to increase vitality and decrease inflammation. Along with the kidneys they are well protected behind the ribs. There are two main sections: the outer and the inner. The outer is the cortex, the main source of most adrenal hormones; the inner is the medulla, the source of adrenaline. The outer cortex is moderated by adrenocorticotropic hormone, ACTH. When the adrenals are under-functioning it goes up, when over-functioning it goes down. ACTH is the hormone from the pituitary gland in the brain, which in turn is influenced by the hypothalamus, an extension of the brain. Our thoughts and feelings have a direct input to its function.

The inner medulla is controlled by thoracic spinal nerves 5-11 of the sympathetic type (the awake-part of the nervous system). It is quickly awakened by a crisis. An old story I recall is how a man actually lifted a car to save the life of a child trapped under it in an accident. In *Les Miserables*, Jean Val Jean is discovered by Javert when he sees him lift a heavy cart off the body of an accident victim. He most likely had a strong surge capacity from his adrenal glands.

The outer part of the adrenal gland, the cortex, consists of three zones: The first one, the outermost, secretes aldosterone that regulates fluid in the body; this is the hormone that a blood pressure medication inhibits to decrease fluid in the body. The second one, the middle layer, secretes **cortisol** and its byproducts that primarily regulate inflammation and provide energy. The third one, the inner layer, secretes **DHEA** and its precursors to testosterone, the androgens or male hormones. Women have some of these too. These hormones especially regulate energy, strength and sexual drive.

The functions of the adrenal gland are best represented by the main hormones of the gland, coritsol and DHEA. They both produce energy and are anti-inflammatory. Cortisol produces energy by tearing down cell activity. DHEA produces energy by building up cell activity and helping to build new cells. These are meant to be in balance and both are important for a dynamic healthy body. Old cells are meant to be torn down and replaced with new cells. Aging occurs as more cells are torn down than are built up. Disease can occur with either one dominating or deficient.

The functions of cortisol are multiple and profound. It increases blood sugar and thus increases energy; although excessive amounts will lead to hyperglycemia, overweight and diabetes. It increases the blood pressure that increases alertness, mood and work capacity; if sustained too long it may lead to hypertension. Cortisol affects the immune system in two ways. It stimulates the immune system that fights bacterial infection. It inhibits the immune system that fights viral infection. It is generally considered an immune inhibitor but has some benefits.

Cortisol decreases inflammation. This is its most well known function because it decreases pain in the joints and muscles from injury, disease and aging. It decreases inflammation from allergies, asthma, chronic obstructive pulmonary disease (COPD) and the intestines. Its anti-inflammatory action is what made cortisol famous in the 1950s and 60s by reversing arthritis, asthma, fatigue and many difficult conditions. Unfortunately, we then discovered its many problems with overuse, meaning high use for periods of several months to years. Those problems are hyperglycemia that leads to diabetes and obesity as well as hypertension and hyperlipidemia, obesity, muscle weakness, cataracts, glaucoma, osteoporosis, earlier memory loss and cancer.

These problems also occur from major prolonged stress, which increases cortisol production more than DHEA, leading to food cravings, especially sweets and processed carbohydrates. These in turn lead to increased weight, blood sugar, elevated blood pressure, weak muscles, thin bones and decreased immune function.

Safe doses of cortisol do not lead to these problems! Cortisol calms us down from major stress. It inhibits the secretion of adrenaline that we pour out when overly upset, worried, frightened or angry. When we get cortisol deficient, the inner adrenal tries to compensate by secreting more adrenaline leading to emotional outbursts.

There are also many benefits to the functions of DHEA. Most of the actions of DHEA are due to its break-down products, its metabolites, especially androstenedione that produces testosterone inside the cell. DHEA is the precursor to many adrenal hormones that increase energy. It stimulates the production of growth hormone in the liver. It also serves as a counter to cortisol, inhibiting its harmful effects and keeping it in balance.

DHEA increases energy, alertness, immune system function and memory. It increases bone density thereby decreasing risk of osteoporosis. DHEA is an anti-oxidant and thus helps cells decrease chemical stress and aging. DHEA also acts on its own in boosting immune system function by stimulating natural killer cell activity. It helps keep blood vessel lining cells (the endothelium) healthy, which decreases hardening of the arteries (arteriosclerosis), and many of the symptoms of aging, especially fatigue and brain function.

Symptoms of adrenal deficiency include fatigue, increased infections and allergies. There may be Intestinal problems, food cravings and food intolerances. Under-functioning adrenals can lead to hair thinning, hair loss, dry skin and dry eyes. Joint pains, especially the low back and neck are common with low adrenal function. There is also the tendency to anxiety, depression and low resistance to stress, including less tolerance to noise. Hypoadrenalism may cause lowered sexual desire, performance and satisfaction. There may even be behavior changes of increased emotionalism, outbursts of anxiety and anger, panic, and other strong verbal retorts.

Cortisol testing can be done by blood, urine or saliva. The usual test that doctors order is blood: an early morning test and/or late afternoon, i.e. Cortisol AM and Cortisol PM. The ACTH challenge test is considered the gold standard but is more cumbersome in requiring one injection and two blood tests, before and after the injection.

The most complete test is the 24-hour urine test. This test measures ten adrenal hormones, nine estrogens and two progesterones, all of which are secreted by the adrenal as well as gender glands. It separates the adrenal hormones into anabolic (building up) hormones and catabolic (breaking down) hormones. The urine test measures the enzymes that influence these reactions and thus provides direction for recommending treatment to adjust them.

Saliva testing for cortisol can be helpful if done over a day long period; i.e. four times during one day. There is a circadian (daily) rhythm to cortisol. It is usually highest in the morning and dips after that. Some people just wake up tired and cannot function for at least a few hours. In these folks cortisol may not be rising fast enough for the early part of the day. These are often the night people, not morning people.

DHEA Sulfate testing is best measured by blood and urine. I find the saliva test to be unreliable; my experience is that it is not accurate for DHEA levels. I have done saliva and blood tests concurrently and found them quite different. For both cortisol and DHEA levels the goal should be in the upper half of normal. Conventional medicine generally recognizes major adrenal deficiency but not mild to moderate deficiency. Major adrenal depletion is Addison's Disease which is associated with major weight loss, profound fatigue and postural dizziness. While Addison's Disease is rare, mild hypoadranlism is relatively common, especially with aging. People feel much better if treated for this condition when warranted.

There are many ways to treat adrenal hypofunction. The first and easiest treatment is whole adrenal extract. It was first used in 1898 by William Osler and was the main form of treatment until the 1950s. Whole adrenal extract is derived from beef adrenal gland. It provides small amounts of all the adrenal cortex hormones and thus a balanced combination. Actual coritsol content is small, about 0.2mg/capsule of hydorcortisone but the effect is still definitely noticeable in many. It is readily available in all health food stores by many companies.

Prescription concentrations of hydrocortisone start at 5mg and a safe amount is 20mg/day. A common prescription is 5mg four times per day although many prescribe 10mg twice per day. Capsules have a tendency to cause heartburn and so should be taken after meals. If patients still have heartburn, I recommend the liquid form. Other adverse effects may include anxiety or difficulty sleeping, especially if taken too late in the day. An occasional person cannot take it later than breakfast time.

The second easiest way to treat low adrenal function is with DHEA. With women the usual dose is 10-25mg depending on blood test and professional advice given. In women under 50, adverse effects may include acne. In women over 50, there is a small chance of adverse effects such as increased risk for facial hair, and loss of scalp hair. Not enough DHEA can cause hair loss and also too much DHEA can cause hair loss; so a balance must be found.

In men the usual dose is 50mg each morning. Depending on results and lab tests the best amount may be 25-100mg. Professional advice is recommended. Adverse effects are may include increased blood pressure, agitated mood and elevated PSA that should be monitored after starting the dose.

The interaction of adrenal hormones with other hormones is important. Both DHEA and whole adrenal should be given at the same time because there is a complementary function; i.e. too much or too little of one will affect production of the other. DHEA will increase the activity of thyroid, estrogen, insulin, testosterone and growth hormone. DHEA will increase receptor sites for estrogen; if the estrogen levels are too low, hot flashes will occur when you start DHEA. If the thyroid is too low, starting DHEA will make it worse. Taking DHEA relieves the pressure of other hormone deficiencies, and optimizing the function of other hormones relieves the strain on the adrenals. The hormone system is ideally treated as a whole symphony with many instruments playing together for high level health.

Estrogens

This is a wonderful hormone and should always be in good supply. There are far more positive benefits than negative. It should be looked on as a powerful healing, energizing hormone. It has potential adverse effects including increasing the risk for cancer, but these are preventable in many ways.

Estrogen has over 400 functions in the body. These are found in five categories: skin, energy, heart, bones and brain.

In the **skin** estrogen decreases wrinkles by increasing connective tissue deposition (collagen) and water content which increase skin thickness and softness. Some women use estriol on the face for this reason.

Energy is a major effect of estrogen and reason enough to begin hormone support. As fatigue is one of the main causes of decreasing quality of life in menopause and peri-menopause this is more than a small contribution to health.

Besides improving energy, estrogen increases longevity by **improving heart risk factors** such as cholesterol, blood pressure, and insulin sensitivity. It decreases LDL, lipoprotein A, and platelet stickiness. It dilates small arteries increasing blood flow and is an anti-oxidant. All these decrease plaque formation and hardening of the arteries and decrease risk of heart disease by about 50%.

Estrogen increases **bone density** by stimulating osteolclasts that recycle bone. Even modest amounts can be effective in treating and preventing osteopenia and osteoporosis.

Estrogen aids many **nerve and brain functions** that increase memory and prevent Alzheimer's syndrome. It increases blood flow, oxygen and glucose levels to the nerves. It boosts NMDA receptors (N-methyl-D-aspartate receptor) by 30%, which is how the nerves communicate with one another, and thus results in increased verbal fluency and memory. As a natural antioxidant it protects nerve cells and nerve growth factor, decreasing chemical changes that lead to Alzheimer's syndrome. Estrogen increases neurotransmitter levels (serotonin and dopamine) leading to increased energy, relaxation and sleep. Most of all estrogen enhances mood and decreases anxiety, irritability and depression by improving nerve hormone supply.

Symptoms of estrogen deficiency occur in the pre-menopausal and early menopausal times. These include hot flashes or facial flushes, more likely but not limited to night time, often resulting in difficulty sleeping. Fatigue is common, especially if sleep is frequently interrupted. Food cravings rise resulting in weight gain especially around the waist. There is increasing risk of brittle hair and nails, thinning of hair and an increase in facial hair. There is thinning of skin resulting in wrinkles, easy bruising and at times oily skin. The urinary and pelvic areas are affected resulting in urinary tract infections, vaginal dryness and vaginal pain with intercourse. Increased headaches and joint pains occur as well as increased blood pressure, cholesterol and diabetes resulting in greater risk for heart attacks. For some there is the increased risk of depression, panic attacks and decreased memory.

There are three main kinds of estrogen: E1, E2 and E3.

E1 is estrone, with one hydroxy, OH group, and the main estrogen in the menopausal state. It is derived from estradiol pre-menopausally from the ovaries and post-menopausally from fat cells. Its primary role is to be a reserve for estradiol if it gets too low.

E2 is estradiol, with two OH groups and the most potent of the three. It is twelve times stronger than E1 and eighty times stronger than E3. Most of the benefits of estrogen come from estradiol. It is especially known to decrease bad cholesterol, triglycerides and fatigue.

E3 is estriol and the main estrogen of pregnancy. It helps restore proper pH of the vagina which benefits the vaginal lining and prevents bladder infections. It decreases cell production in the breast, uterus and ovaries and therefore helps decrease the risk for cancer. Estriol also decreases LDL cholesterol and increases HDL cholesterol but not as strongly as estradiol, and thus it doesn't help as much with the heart, bones, and brain.

There are many ways to test estrogen levels. The most common way to test estrogens is the blood. It is readily available with the local labs, but there are potential complications. In peri-menopause, the levels fluctuate easily during the month creating wide swings of levels, complicating assessment and treatment. The recommended time to test estrogen is one week after menstruation begins or one week before menstruation. After menopause, which is one year without a cycle, the levels are more steady and only a problem if changing hormones doses within 4-6 weeks before testing.

Saliva is used by a growing number of practitioners. I have not been satisfied with its consistency but some physicians use it confidently. It is easy to do, self administered and inexpensive although insurance is less likely to cover it.

The most comprehensive test is the 24-hour urine test. It measures ten different kinds of estrogen. Blood tests only measure estradiol. The urine test measures estrone (E1), estradiol (E2), and estriol (E3). It also measures hydoxy estrogens and methyl estrogens. The methyl estrogens are less affected by cancer and so more desirable. (If there are too many hydroxyl estrogens they can be shifted by diet, supplements and medication). The test also measures two types of hydoxy estrogens, 2 and 16. The 2 estrogen may be more beneficial because it is less likely to convert to cancer risk and the 16 type is less beneficial because it is more likely to increase cell changes toward cancer. (These concentrations can also be shifted by diet and supplements). This test can be done to assess risk for cancer and should be considered by more women. It is not a guarantee of cancer protection and should not be considered a substitute for routine breast exams and mammograms.

Topical estrogen in the form of a patch or cream is the healthiest way to use it. The patches are covered by insurance and are placed on the skin 1-2 times per week. A common cream formula is biestrogen: 80% estriol and 20% estradiol. The topical forms are best because the estrogen then doesn't pass through the liver in large amounts and thereby decreases the risk of venous thrombophlebitis.

Some practitioners are recommend intravaginal or vulvar cream to follow nature's natural blood collection pathway for estrogen. The creams require compounding formulas. The advantages are a greater precision of dose for individual use as well as having the option to add a variety of other hormones to the mixture. At times it is appropriate and convenient to prescribe estriol with estradiol, as well as progesterone and testosterone. DHEA and pregnenolone can be added as well. Although compounding allows for greater individualizing doses and combinations insurance companies may not cover them.

My experience with estrogen replacement for menopause is that 25% of women have no problem with menopause; 50% respond quite well to initial treatment, and 25% have difficulty. The more complicated conditions may need multiple attempts to adjust the dosages. In addition they may need a more comprehensive hormone approach that includes thyroid, adrenal and pituitary hormones. Often they are also more likely to need a healthy lifestyle of excellent diet, exercise and stress management. Of course, all of these should be the goal of each of us for the best of health, optimal vitality and longevity with quality years, not just quantity. The 25% who do not need hormone replacement at the time of menopause may require hormone support later. Their adrenal glands adjust readily but become deficient eventually. Some women can go for many years without hormone replacement.

Oral estrogen in pill and capsule form have several potential adverse effects. These include increased carbohydrate cravings and subsequent weight gain. In addition there is a decrease in the formation of tryptophan and serotonin metabolism resulting in less calmness and happiness. Oral doses increase liver enzyme strain and the risk for gallstones. They lower growth hormone supply by 50% and may increase blood pressure and triglycerides. Topical prescriptions are much less likely to have adverse effects.

Progesterone

Progesterone is produced in the ovaries and the adrenal glands. During the reproductive years in women, progesterone is secreted in its highest concentrations the last 2 weeks of the monthly menstrual cycle. The levels peak about one week before menstruation. When the levels start to decrease menstruation is set to begin. Progesterone is produced in men in much smaller amounts by the adrenal glands.

Progesterone promotes health and healing in many ways. It produces a natural calming effect that enhances sleep and counters depression. It lowers blood pressure, cholesterol, and inflammation. It increases scalp hair, libido, and bone strength. It improves metabolism, immunity and nerve protection.

Progesterone increases the energy level by providing precursor hormones to the adrenal glands. Of the 150 hormones produced in the adrenals most are derived from progesterone especially including testosterone and aldosterone, a fluid-regulating hormone. Progesterone also increases energy levels by enhancing thyroid function.

Cancer protection is one of progesterone's many functions. Estrogen increases the number of cells in the breasts, ovaries and uterus. Progesterone matures these cells. Cancer cells are more likely to result from abnormalities of cell reproduction during the early phase of their life span, called the juvenile state. When matured beyond this state they are less likely to become destructive cancer cells.

There are symptoms of progesterone loss. These include weight gain, headaches, fatigue and inflammation. Premenstrual symptoms in the form of pain, anxiety, depression and irritability are often a progesterone deficiency condition.

The main cause of low progesterone is impaired production. This often begins in the early 40s in most women. Other causes include an excessive intake of sugary, fatty foods and deficiencies of Vitamins A, B6, and C. Low thyroid function and anti-depressants may also lower progesterone function. One of the most potent causes is physical and emotional stress. Initially stress increases the amounts of progesterone secreted but then leads to a subsequent deficiency.

Progestins are synthetic non-bioidentical forms of progesterone. These are alien to our body's healthy function. The Women's Health Study that caused a major change in hormone replacement therapy use implicated progestins as the main cause of increasing breast cancer prevalence. They were initially found to decrease uterine cancer in women taking estrogen for hormone replacement. They did decrease uterine cancer but increased the risk for breast cancer. Progestins also have many other adverse effects including nausea, vomiting, fatigue, depression and irritability.

Excessive bioidentical progesterone has ill effects, too. There may be increased appetite that leads to food cravings and fat storage, which leads to increased cholesterol, triglycerides and insulin resistance, all of which lead to increased weight. There may be increased depression, fatigue and decreased libido. Progesterone increases relaxation of pelvic ligaments that may cause back and joint pains. Increased relaxation of the intestines may lead to bloating and constipation. The goal is always balance, the right amount for your body, and that varies from one to another.

Progesterone treatment is usually in the form of a cream or capsule. Over the counter creams are 3%, meaning 30mg/gram, a modest amount for replacement. Compounded creams can vary depending on the prescription from smaller to full therapeutic amounts. There is a great deal of controversy about how much progesterone is healthy. The amount needed depends on the goal. Small amounts are sufficient for basic needs of many women. However, larger amounts are needed when the goal is to establish a continuing menstrual cycle. At times, larger capsule amounts are used to enhance sleep, as byproducts of progesterone produced in the liver promote sedating effects on the nervous system.

Progesterone treatment is designed for specific benefits. It may improve adrenal function as a precursor to many adrenal hormones and the vitality that may ensue. It may relax the body and enhance sleep. Or it may be used to balance larger amounts of estrogen used in major hormone replacement to diminish excess energy or the risk of cancer.

Testosterone for Men and Women

There are many benefits of testosterone in men and women. Although primarily known as a male hormone, women produce it, too, and for important reasons. Testosterone is an energy hormone; it vitalizes many functions of the body especially the muscular system, noticeable when associated with a vigorous exercise routine that includes some weight lifting. The heart is a muscle and, not surprisingly, it responds well to optimizing testosterone levels; men live longer who have higher levels than those who do not although research on this is controversial. It is a longevity hormone for men and women for multiple reasons besides the heart. It decreases bone deterioration and increases muscle mass, tone and strength. It elevates norepinephrine resulting in improved memory, emotional well-being and self confidence.

Dr. Farid Saab reported a recent study at the 2012 annual meeting of the endocrine society. His group studied 255 men over five years with hypogonadism defined as a total testosterone of less than 350ng/dL. Ninety per cent lost over 10 pounds and 97% decreased the waist circumference by 10cm or more. 76% lost over 20 pounds, 53% lost over 30 pounds and 31% lost 45 pounds. The study also showed that testosterone increased fat free mass, meaning muscle mass. Participants were not placed on a special diet or exercise regimen.

Testosterone is especially known for its effect on the sexual impulse and performance. It increases sexual interest in many, though not all; it may take up to six months for a full effect. Men usually take testosterone on a daily basis or every other week if by injection.

Women usually take testosterone on a cyclic basis or as needed. The ovaries secrete larger amounts a few days before ovulation and a few days before menstruation. Supplementing during these times can improve nature's cycle. It can also be used for a few days prior to or on the day of potential sexual activity. Some women use it on the clitoris just before sexual activity.

Symptoms of testosterone deficiency include weight gain, fatigue, anxiety, and decreased libido. Less known symptoms of deficiency are skin changes, abdominal fat, and memory loss. The cutaneous changes are dry thin skin, thinning hair, sagging cheeks and thin lips.

It is important to know the causes of low testosterone. The most common ones are aging, menopause, stress, depression, burnout and psychological trauma. Medications that cause testosterone depletion are statins, birth control pills and chemotherapy.

There are some conditions that are aggravated by low testosterone. These include diabetes, metabolic syndrome, heart disease, Alzheimer's syndrome and cancer, all of which improve with treatment.

Testosterone can be measured by blood and urine tests. Blood tests are the easiest; all labs do this. Until recently, the normal value for women was 0-80 though I can't imagine why 0 is okay. Lately the range has been given as 4-45. My goal is to see it in the upper half of normal. After starting treatment I pay attention to the response of treatment to find the optimal dose.

For men and women there is a free and total testosterone panel. The free portion means unbound to protein; the free form is the most active form and a better way to assess full function. Again the goal is the upper half of normal.

Urine tests can also be done. The 24-hour urine test is an excellent way to measure testosterone because the window of assessment is longer. Some labs will also offer a panel of multiple adrenal, androgen (testosterone) and estrogen levels with the same specimen. The urine panel is the most comprehensive way to evaluate testosterone and its many metabolites.

Testosterone treatment has several options. In women my first choice is DHEA. In 70% of women it will increase testosterone by using 5-25mg per day. The second choice is to use testosterone cream. It may be added to estrogen and/or progesterone cream. I usually start with a modest amount, i.e. 0.5-2mg/day; it can be increased slowly up to 10mg/day, though most prefer modest amounts to avoid adverse effects.

The unusual way for women to increase testosterone is to get it from the husband. I had a woman patient whose levels were terribly high and we could not figure it out until we realized that her husband put his testosterone cream on at bedtime. It was being transferred to his wife from skin to skin contact.

For men the options are different. Cream is the most physiologic, i.e. closest to what the body produces on a daily basis. A sublingual troche can be used but it dissolves slowly, so is a bit annoying. The easiest, most noticeable and least expensive form of testosterone is the injection form. It is usually given every other week although some find that a weekly dose works best. Men who take testosterone need to have follow-up blood tests to be sure the dose doesn't go too high which increases adverse effects and may increase prostate specific antigen, the PSA.

Besides taking testosterone directly it can be increased in other ways. Testosterone increases with weight loss, exercise and increasing sleep. Increasing precursor proteins such as arginine, leucine and glutamine may improve testosterone levels. Zinc supplementation may also help.

Excess testosterone causes trouble too. Adverse effects may include hypertension, increased sexual drive, anxiety, depression, agitation and anger. There may be salt and sugar cravings that lead to weight gain. Women are more prone to acne, especially in those under 50 years of age. In older women there is a greater tendency for hair loss and new facial hair. Insulin resistance and increased heart disease risk are long term problems that occur with larger doses. There is no clear evidence that testosterone causes or increases the risk of prostate cancer, although the fear is great.

Growth Hormone

The pituitary gland is situated in the upper brain behind the middle of the forehead. It is often referred to as the master gland because its secretions stimulate most of the other hormone glands. It is the source of thyroid stimulating hormone (TSH), adrenocorticotropic hormone (ACTH, which stimulates the adrenal glands), follicle stimulating hormone (FSH, stimulating the ovaries for ovulation), and luteinizing hormone (LH, stimulating the uterine lining for menstruation or pregnancy). All of these hormones are in turn stimulated by releasing factor hormones from the hypothalamus, an extension of the brain right above the pituitary gland.

Growth hormone is a major hormone secreted by the pituitary gland. As with all hormones, growth hormone secretion declines with age, although it continues to have the potential for stimulation longer than the other hormone systems. Levels decline with age as the growth hormone releasing factors from the hypothalamus diminish. Somatopause is the name given to the decline of growth hormone in aging adults.

Symptoms of growth hormone deficiency affect many organs of the body. Wrinkles appear on the skin because of the loss of pro-collagen (it is a connective tissue glue-like substance that preserves the integrity of the skin). Decreasing levels of growth hormone leads to more wrinkles, loss of nail and hair growth. It may also cause dehydration due to reduced kidney blood flow and less efficient re-absorption of fluid in their filtering units. These in turn result in thinning of the skin and depletion of bone tissue. Loss of growth hormone decreases muscle function including the heart, the most important muscle of the body. In addition, lipid levels of the various types of cholesterol are adversely affected, and this also increases the risk for cardiovascular degeneration. Growth hormone affects metabolism and thus diminishing amounts result in less energy production and more fatigue. Growth hormone deficiency results in less blood sugar entering the cells (hypoglycemia), more fat deposition resulting in higher unhealthy weight (total body and abdominal fat), thyroid inhibition and less protein production. All of these condtions implicate growth hormone loss with decreased energy, quality of life and sense of well-being.

The main test for growth hormone is IGF-1 which is Insulin-like Growth Factor 1. Growth hormone acts like insulin in that it enhances entry of blood sugar into the cell. IGF-1 is a breakdown product of growth hormone and a more stable way to measure growth hormone levels. Growth hormone itself is released in bursts throughout the day and is therefore very difficult to measure accurately. It is uncommon for older adults to have below normal levels of IGF-1, but common to have values in the lower half levels of normal which should be considered suboptimal. Most laboratories lower the range of normal as we age making it more difficult to establish guidelines for optimal function tests. As with the other hormone systems, it is necessary to ask what is optimal as opposed to abnormal or deficient. Results should always be correlated with symptoms of deficiency and, at times, response to treatment.

Many studies have been conducted verifying the values of growth hormone treatment. Over one hundred years ago it was used on children of very slow growth. Most studies began after 1958 when it was synthesized and more readily used in treatment research. The first prominent study was reported in the *New England Journal of Medicine.* It was conducted on 12 healthy individuals and showed in them an increase in muscle mass, bone density and skin thickness; fat tissue decreased by over 14%.

Subsequent studies show that growth hormone improves the function of most organs of the body. It increases muscle strength and stamina with improved heart pump action. It stimulates bones by increasing osteoblast formation, the cells that produce new bone. It improves intestinal function, sexual drive and performance, hair growth and color, vision, and sleep. It improves the immune system and wound healing. It also enhances nerve function by improving memory and mood.

The most well known way to treat growth hormone deficiency is with growth hormone. But because of its instability in the intestinal tract, it must be given by injection, one or more times per day. It is expensive for most people.

Growth hormone has a long list of potential adverse effects. These may include cancer, carpal tunnel, edema, heart disease, hypoglycemia, hyperglycemia, decreased insulin sensitivity, and intestinal disturbances.

Fortunately there are many ways to improve growth hormone secretion. Diet, exercise and other hormones can have a positive impact. A poor diet and obesity diminish growth hormone secretion. Intense exercise and fasting increase it as do estrogen and testosterone replacement.

The greatest capacity for increasing growth hormone safely and expensively is with supplements. The most important are the amino acid protein building blocks. The main one is arginine, although glutamine and ornithine also play a role. These effects are aided by niacin (B3), calcium, magnesium, potassium and zinc. The amounts vary with different company products. As these are primarily protein supplements they are most potent when taken alone without food, i.e. one hour before food or two hours after.

The most intriguing potential stimulants of growth hormone are the nerve hormones acetyl choline and dopamine. Both have been shown to increase growth hormone and are themselves increased by taking the amino acid precursors choline and tyrosine.

Unfortunately, supplements are unlikely to have a major effect on hormone levels.

Neurotransmitter Hormones

Nerve hormones are finally getting some attention. In the recent past, many studies have documented the effects of neurotransmitters on mood disorders, especially depression and anxiety. A variety of antidepressants have been developed, and they do aid many people in many ways. Now there are newer, innovative uses of neurotransmitters.

The function of nerve hormones is to transmit information through the nervous system. The nervous system consists of sensory nerves (sight, hearing, touch, taste and smell), the voluntary muscle system (that allows motion and action) and the autonomic nerve system (for automatic functions like heart rate, respiration, digestion and elimination). Each nerve consists of a receiving end and a transmitting end. One nerve communicates with the next nerve by sending an electrical impulse to the transmitting end, stimulating the nerve ending, which discharges nerve hormones. When a critical number of impulses reaches the next nerve an impulse is generated. Nerve endings communicate by nerve hormones not by direct contact.

The external purpose of the nervous system is to transmit awareness of the world outside, access memories, thoughts and feelings that relate to it, and communicate these for interpretation, understanding and action. The internal purpose is to be a vehicle of expressing our innate intelligence, stability, creative responsiveness and energy.

There are over 150 different neurotransmitters. The well-recognized ones are melatonin, serotonin, dopamine and adrenaline. Problems occur with overuse and depletion. Serotonin has been shown to affect appetite, arousal, temperature regulation, sensory perception, sleep, emotion and mood and reward perception. Dopamine function affects cognitive control, working memory, mood, motivation, motor system function, reward perception and sexual arousal. Noradrenaline affects wakefulness and attention, circadian rhythm, cognitive control, working memory, hunger, respiration, negative emotional memory and reward perception. Adrenaline affects neurotransmitter and adrenal hormones leading to fight or flight and subsequent increased heart rate, blood pressure, blood sugar, muscle action and fear.

Symptoms of neurotransmitter depletion include depression, anxiety, fatigue, insomnia, lack of concentration and decreased memory. The reason nerve hormones become depleted is because they are overused, aging and congenital predispositions to lower levels.

More innovative uses of neurotransmitters began in weight loss programs several years ago. Initially in many of these clinics weight loss medications were used. When Fenfluramine was found to be associated with pulmonary hypertension, antidepressants began to be used. Eventually a few began to experiment with precursor amino acids to perform the same function of the medications. The protein building blocks of the neurotransmitters were found to be very effective.

A number of medical conditions were found to improve from the use of neurotransmitter precursor proteins. Depression became one of them. The precursor proteins build up the amount of nerve hormone levels. The antidepressants improve delivery from one nerve ending to the next but do not improve the amount available. The other conditions found to be helped include ADD, insomnia, obesity, anxiety, migraine headaches, premenstrual syndrome, fibromyalgia, chronic fatigue, adrenal fatigue, chronic pain, irritable bowel syndrome, and cognitive deterioration.

Testing is not reliable until full amounts of the amino acids are in use. At that point spot urine tests may be beneficial for fine-tuning amounts used.

For treatment I recommend the amino acids combinations of tyrosine and 5 hydoxy- tryptamine. Ideally these need to be in a 10:1 ratio. These must be taken together as they compete for the same enzyme, aromatic amino acid decarboxylase, for the synthesis of serotonin and dopamine. Taking 5 HTP without tyrosine will cause a depletion of dopamine, and tyrosine without 5 HTP will cause a depletion of serotonin. At times it may be necessary to monitor neurotransmitter levels with follow-up urine tests after reaching full amounts.

Lifestyle Effects on Hormone Levels

Healthy nutrition enhances the function of every hormone system in the body. You can be sure an unhealthy diet limits optimal secretion. The usual good food is necessary: a rich array of vegetables, raw more than cooked; lean meats, especially fish and fowl, preferably range fed; modest amounts of whole fruit, not juice; avoiding most of the sweet, salty sumptuous shelves of processed foods and drinks. Optimal protein is essential.

Exercise also plays a role. By increasing heart pump power there are a larger number of blood vessels reaching every winding nook and cranny, cell and organ in the body. Work-out sweat and tears increase oxygen absorption and waste removal ensuring less chemical interference with the many vital functions of our hormone function.

Sunlight has been documented to enhance hormone function. Zane Kime, M.D., wrote a book many years ago called *Sunlight Could Save Your Life*. He listed many references to how sunlight striking the body increases hormone production of every hormone in the body. The more skin exposed to the light the more hormone secretion is stimulated, especially the adrenal and gender hormones.

Vitamin D has the structure and function of a hormone and is now being newly categorized as such by a growing number of researchers. The last few years has seen a whole new emphasis on studies of vitamin D. There is a growing list of its many benefits to the body. It is being shown to not only strengthen bone but also muscle and immune capacity. Early studies are finding links with low levels of D and higher incidence of breast and prostate cancer.

The role of attitude and hormones deserves some attention. If our mood can obviously affect muscle tension and intestinal activity surely it is directly connected to hormone secretion and interaction. I do know that when we are younger with full hormone supplies surging through the body, we respond fully and usually excessively to fears, doubts and worries. There are many references to how stress leads to higher levels of each of the major hormone systems. Hyperthyroidism and hypercortisolism are two good examples. However over time the glands wear out leading to under functioning secretions resulting in fatigue and many other symptoms. Healthy hormone function must include attention to healthy moods and attitudes. Choosing cheerfulness instead of sadness, graciousness instead of grief, goodwill instead of anger, and enthusiasm instead of remorseful regrets surely adds energy to every hormone system in the body.

Chapter 7

Healing Pain Leads to Wholeness

One of the most dramatic lessons in mobilizing healing power came out of my work with chronic pain patients. Working at Dr. Shealy's Chronic Pain Clinic for over four years, I learned a great deal about what it is, where it comes from and how to heal it. By the time patients came to us they had been in chronic pain an average of four years. They averaged three operations for pain relief and were addicted to pain relief medications. They were depressed and in dysfunctional marriage and family relationships. They were surgical and medical failures. However, in our program, most of them succeeded in lessening pain considerably. Those who were most likely to heal followed the suggestions we taught and re-awakened their healing centers. Our goal was to work on healing the physical, emotional and mental issues, exposing and healing the past and the present. It worked for those who pursued a comprehensive program of healing. First I want to explain a little more about the experience of pain.

Pain is the initial warning sign of danger or damage. A whole organ system is dedicated to protecting the body with nerve endings for pain detection. The skin system is an extension of the nervous system, a built-in sensing alarm activated at the least sign of invasion or harm. We are highly sophisticated organisms of chemicals and organs that are very vulnerable to injury. We are a soup of chemicals that can spill easily. The same nerve endings that line the skin also line each organ of the body. To prevent damage we must pay attention to the warning signs and trace them back to the source.

Pain is experienced in the body at three different levels of the nervous system: the skin, the midbrain and the higher brain. The skin sensation nerve endings that register pain are where most people notice injury or strain. The skin nerve fibers send signals along the nerves to the spine, from where it moves along distinct fiber networks integrated in the middle of the brain, the thalamus part of the brain. From there it is intertwined with the emotion centers of the brain. The third level of pain perception is within the thinking part of the brain, the frontal cortex, through which we express intelligence, insight, and meaning, which is big picture context to pain.

Pain needs to be considered as a function of one or more of these levels of experience. The more we can engage meaning, the less likely the pain will interfere with our life and its purposes. When we suffer severe pain we may well need to consult with the professionals available, but we can also engage our body, mind and higher self to expose what is missing and what will lead to healing.

Healing Acute Muscle Pain

There are many kinds of muscle pain because there are many muscles attaching to many bones in different ways. Even though I am a strong advocate of healthy aging medicine, it has become quite clear that we are more susceptible to muscle strain as we age. We injury more easily, take longer to heal and do not heal as completely.

A 54-year-old woman came in to see me recently. She was very concerned about a new pain in the groin areas on the insides of the hips. It was an unusual pain for her though she felt something like this a few years ago for a short period of time. Over the counter Ibuprofen was not helpful. Prescription Tramadol at 2-3 times/day was not helpful enough. She was scheduled to take a much-anticipated trip to Europe within just a few weeks and was worried whether she would be able to walk enough to enjoy the trip. No matter how well such a trip is planned, it requires much walking, standing and waiting in unfamiliar territory. Pain is the last thing you want to take with you on a major trip.

I questioned and examined her. It was quite apparent that she had an inguinal groin tendonitis from muscle strain. There was no sign of nerve damage, back disc damage or blood clots in the legs. I reassured her about the nature of these problems but was puzzled about the cause. With persistent questions she finally admitted to driving more than usual in making preparations for all the special purchases needed for the trip. She was reluctant to believe that driving more would trigger such discomfort but was satisfied with further discussion that such could be the case. She healed quickly and had a wonderful trip.

We need to become experts at coaching ourselves through the problems that arise. Diagnosis of a relatively minor problem heals our fear of something worse. Much of the healing we do in medicine is reassurance that you don't have something serious, like heart disease, nerve damage or cancer. When we know the problem is not serious we can stop worrying and use the energy in better ways. We can more easily pursue tasks at hand for upcoming events, knowing that the body can heal. Fear spoils much of the enjoyment available to us.

Treatment for minor muscle strain includes the proper use of ice packs. Ice is always better with muscle strain during the first 48 hours because it decreases blood flow and thereby decreases leaking from injured blood vessels, limiting the size of a bruise. Ice also shuts down pain nerve fibers, at least temporarily. After the first few days heat or ice may be used. The heat can accelerate healing by increasing blood flow and delivery of immune system nutrients that promote the healing process. After the first forty-eight hours I encourage experimenting to find out which works best.

Physical treatment options for acute pain should include the following:

1. Ice (the first 48 hours).
2. Heat (after the first 48 hours if it feels better).

3. Gentle stretching.
4. Self massage (around the area of injury rather than directly on it).
5. Deep tissue massage (the type is not as important as the skill and trust in the practitioner).
6. Physical therapy (for assessment and treatment, especially massage and muscle strengthening).
7. Spinal adjustment (Chiropractic or Osteopathic).
8. Acupuncture (with or without electrical stimulation).
9. Topical creams (herbal, homeopathic, medicinal and prescription).
10. Over the counter medications (Ibuprofen, Aspirin, Tylenol).
11. Prescription medication if needed (analgesic, anti-inflammatory, muscular relaxants).
12. Injections of Novocain, Cortisone or Proliferant medications.
13. Seek professional help if worried or not responding to basic treatments.
14. Assess the cause, learn from the event, encourage self-healing and be grateful for the efforts being made.

Emotional aspects play a role in acute pain injuries. Often I ask what was going on before the injury. Although accidents occur, many are the result of distraction due to emotional distress. At the Pain Clinic one day I gave a talk on the cause of accidents. I discussed experiences of people who had increased their risk for accidents by their fear, frustration and worry. As I was talking I saw a sheriff approach the building. He was gone before I finished the talk. Right after the talk I spoke with the secretary who visited with him. Earlier in the morning, at the beginning of the day's session, the husband of a patient bumped into another patient's car, leading to a call to the sheriff.

The coincidence was not lost on me. I tracked down the driver of the car and asked him how things were going. Without much prompting, it became apparent that he was quite upset with the clinic because we were not relieving the pain of his wife fast enough. We discussed the situation further and the options available for her, and she did improve during her stay. But the confirmation of stress as cause of the accident was reassuring and hopefully helpful to many who have heard the story.

Most accidents are not accidental. As we get emotionally distressed we are more easily distracted, less attentive and more vulnerable to accidents. The mental component of pain is the context in which it occurs. The cause and sequence of events are not often clear or definitive. But the feelings and thoughts we have create circumstances that set events in motion. Learning how to confront crises as quickly as possible may prevent many more problems from happening.

Healing Major Chronic Pain

Chronic pain is one of the most debilitating conditions we experience. It is all absorbing, debilitating and depressing. We all feel it at some time but for many it is totally disabling. Fortunately, pain can be the trigger we need to learn what we need to know and find the strength to use it.

At the Pain Clinic we offered a thorough medical evaluation, frequent therapeutic massage, gentle spinal adjustment, practical acupuncture, extensive counseling and neurological reprogramming. The most effective part of the program was the nerve retraining through mental exercises.

Assessment of a chronic pain condition requires a thorough review of what preceded the onset. This includes a complete history of symptoms, triggering events, progression, treatments tried and responses. At the clinic we used a pain profile of five categories (0-100, 100 being the worse end of the extreme) measuring average pain intensity (100 is passing out), limitation of physical activity (100 is unable to get out of bed), per cent of time pain is felt (100 is every waking moment), affect on mood (100 is not wanting to live anymore) and medication intake (100 is physical addiction).

Following a review of the physical state, ideally there is psychological review of emotional status. This includes an assessment of the fear, doubt, guilt and anger present; the need for forgiveness, insight and inspiration; the current state of the capacity to express goodwill, gratitude and meaningful activity. This will also include a review of major relationships, the impact of pain and unfulfilled expectations.

It became quite apparent at the pain clinic that most of the patients had a long history of emotional pain. There were stories of some physical abuse in childhood. More common was a family history of emotional neglect, abuse, and, at times, abandonment. Most often we found that life stress events triggered injury or illness that began the chronic pain condition.

Acupuncture Heals Pain

I first heard about acupuncture when in medical school. It sounded intriguing and safe if it worked. I saw it done when visiting the Edgar Cayce medical research clinic in Phoenix AZ. While waiting to meet the physician head of the clinic, I heard a nurse report to a family member in the waiting room, that it would be a little longer wait "because it took more time than planned to balance the meridians." I did not know what that meant but was very intrigued to find out.

Eventually I became a medical resident at the clinic and witnessed several acupuncture treatments. However, I did not study it carefully until joining the Pain Clinic. Dr. Shealy taught me how to perform acupuncture for pain relief. He took a very pragmatic approach to it, focusing treatment on the areas of pain and tenderness. It worked in many patients to the point where we observed that acupuncture initially helped relieve pain up to 90% of the time. My observation was that it had a major impact on about 50% of our patients and a dramatic effect on a few.

I am convinced that acupuncture should be a common treatment modality for all specialties with chronic pain patients. Acupuncture is the art of using needles to penetrate the skin to promote healing. The art is thousands of years old and developed in China. Jesuit priests studied it carefully in the 16th century when visiting China and brought it to France and Europe. it now is practiced all over the world but only widely for the last 50 years in large part due to President Nixon's opening relations with China in 1972.

Chinese acupuncturists developed a complex system of meridians, lines of energy. These start or end at the head, hands, feet and spine. Along these lines are points of tension, higher points of energy that affect the flow of Chi, the energy of vitality. When the proper points are treated, the energy flows more freely, resulting in restoration of optimal function. There are many points and combinations of points that one learns with training and experience. Interestingly, many of the meridians do follow the paths of major nerve branches, especially in the arms and legs

The first time I did acupuncture was for a woman in her 30s. She had a right shoulder injury due to lifting boxes at work. After two years of physical therapy, injections and medications, she was still in pain, without relief. She was reluctant to have acupuncture or needles of any kind. However, she finally agreed to a "few needle treatments." I inserted one needle in the mid upper shoulder region, at the midway point between the top of the shoulder and the neck. Within minutes she began to notice relief. She subsequently reported complete relief requiring no further treatments. Follow-up exams revealed no tenderness or limitation of movement.

I have continued to use acupuncture on many patients since leaving the pain clinic. As I pursued my Family Practice work, I often offer acupuncture to those with chronic pain conditions. Many chose the treatments and most find them helpful.

Most physicians and nurses can easily receive basic treatment principles. It is safer than all prescription and over-the-counter medications. Acupuncture should be available for those with chronic headaches, back and neck pain, abdominal conditions, menstrual pain conditions, post herpetic neuralgia (shingles) and cancer pain. There is rationale for performing acupuncture on a wide range of diseases other than pain with appropriate evaluation and examination.

When I do acupuncture, I usually include suggestions for relaxation and healing affirmation. After needle insertion and adjusting to the needling, I lower the lights to induce a state of relaxation. I suggest the calling forth of an experience in nature, a pleasant memory or time of comfort. I suggest the patient to quietly consider the following questions: "Why do I need to be well? Why do I deserve to be well? What will I do with the healing I receive?" This sequence of questions seems to be helpful to many as it invokes the will-to-heal and the energy that accompanies it.

Nerve Retraining

Neurological retraining is the process of retraining nerves to transmit normal sensations instead of pain. Once the diagnosis has ruled out infection, tumor or a surgical condition the pain is not longer of any value. The nerves need retaining. This is done primarily through a series of mental exercises that progress form simple relaxation to advanced levels of visualization and meditation.

There are many types of relaxation-insight exercises. The initial goal is to find one that works, that consistently creates a deep sense of being relaxed and yet awake. In this state there is usually a deep sense of comfort without pain. In this state the body is more receptive to creative suggestions for healing. These suggestions may take the form of reverent music, soothing colors and positive experiences in nature.

During the relaxed state it is also more possible to suggest insight questions to promote healing fear, frustration, worry, anger, guilt and grief. To heal fear we invoke courage and strength by recalling prior success and larger than life people who are important to us. To heal frustration we invoke calmness and confidence by recalling experiences of handling stress well. To heal anger we review the value of being forgiven for our own mistakes and misjudgments. To heal guilt we contemplate the compassion of la loving parent or friend who accepts us in spite of our misdeeds of neglect. To heal grief we express gratitude for what we have and the small gifts of kindness wherever we see them.

As we create positive sensations of enjoyment, comfort and acceptance of self we retrain nerves to relax and calm down. We learn how to breathe new life into all of who we are. It changes how we feel and think about ourself and consider worthwhile possibilities for our life in spite of limitations.

At the pain clinic we had a high success rate. 84% of those attending a 12 day session had greater than 50% relief of chronic pain at the end of the program. About 70% of those following the lifestyle changes recommended were successfully relieving pain one year later. Most patients markedly decreased the use of pain relieving medication, increased physical activity and rejuvenated major relationships. Nerve s can be reprogrammed with a sincere, persistent intention to do the healing work required.

Affirmations Heal Pain

Chronic pain is usually the result of a long history of disappointing physical and psychological events. We found that extensive counseling could reverse many of these old patterns. One of the counseling tools we used was the creation and use of healing affirmations.

Sandra was a woman in her mid-30s with two young children. She had low back pain for two years that was not responding to medications, physical therapy or exercise suggestions. She had declined surgery but was in continuous daily pain. When asked how the pain interfered with her life, she became tearful, recalling an afternoon when her young daughter came to her, pulled on her dress and asked "Why don't you play with us like you used to." She could not do the housework and certainly could not be the wife she wanted to be. However, when asked what activity she would most like to do when she became well, she immediately said, "Riding my motorcycle." This used to be a common event she shared with her husband before the back pain began.

She described the feeling of riding her motorcycle that became the source of her healing affirmation. She created the phrase "I am excited, exhilarated, happy and healthy." She was advised to use these words, picturing herself motorcycling down a favorite road, and to do so every hour of the day for at least five minutes. At the end of the two-week session she was about 50% better. I received a letter from her six weeks after leaving the clinic with a picture of her on a motorcycle. She had just returned from a 1,500-mile motorcycle ride with her husband, each on their own motorcycle. She was feeling great, healthy and free of pain. I am sure her relief came more from her willingness to focus frequently on her positive healing affirmation than anything else we tried.

There are many ways to form healing affirmations. The simple way is to choose an image of health that is desired, preferably an activity that requires full use of the body. This can be a memory of when the body worked well at an enjoyable and/or meaningful activity with friends or family. Visualize it and then describe it to yourself. What words describe it well? Choose those and create a phrase in the present tense. A short, simple phrase is easiest to remember and use.

The next step is to energize it with why you need to be well, and why you need to be able to do this activity healthy and well. This step usually requires a sincere appeal for help from deep within. Then it is necessary to plug into a source of power that will energize the healing requested. This is done by recalling a prior peak experience of love, joy or having done the right thing at the right time.

The final step is to practice it often: attune to the source of life, the image of the activity chosen and the words that describe it. This must be practiced with full expectation of positive results, at least five minutes three times per day for one month. Examples can be: "I am healthy and well, calm and confident." "I feel strong, flexible and comfortable." "I am relaxed, happy and healthy in every way."

The history of healing affirmations goes back to the beginning of time or at least to recent ancient times. Sacred texts have often been used as seed thoughts and feelings for what we need to replace what is distressing or missing. Psalms, prayers and appeals for healing are old traditions that have grown over time. Emil Coue, a French psychologist and pharmacist, popularized the use of healing phrases in the late 1800s. His most well known phrase became, "Every day in every way I am getting better and better."

Chronic Pain Healing Options

1. **Ice and/or heat**, up to 20 minutes/hour; ice is necessary for the first 48 hours after an injury, however, after this time, whichever feels better and relieves pain best should be used. The ice works by decreasing nerve action; heat works by increasing blood flow that delivers immune repair cells and chemicals of healing.

2. **Exercise is essential and at times the most important tool for relief of pain and healing.** Stretching exercises done slowly and easily is necessary for recovery. Although most people need some guidance, a regular routine can usually be pursued effectively.
3. More vigorous exercise is not usually possible in most chronic pain conditions, but some **aerobic exercise** routine may be very helpful. Those who have at least a walking routine heal faster. Swimming is probably safer for most because the body weight is supported by the water instead of the spine so that more vigorous exercise is better tolerated.
4. **An anti-inflammatory diet** may also be helpful. It is known that arachidonic acid will increase inflammation and that a diet without it may decrease inflammation. Red meats and dairy have higher amounts of arachidonic acid than fish and fowl. Range-fed chickens and beef have higher amounts of omega 3 fatty acids that have anti-inflammatory effects on the body. Of course, optimal weight ensures less pressure on many joints of the body, especially the low back.
5. **A transcutaneous electrical neurostimulator** (TENS) unit is a small battery device (usually 9 volt) that often relieves acute and chronic pain. At the pain clinic we found that every patient initially had some relief with a TENS unit. At the end of a 2-week session, about 50% of patients purchased one for home use, and half of those continued to have benefit over the long term. I think every home should have a TENS unit available. Amazon has an effective inexpensive device.
6. There are a wide range of **nutritional supplements** that have some pain relieving abilities. The ones that decrease inflammation (fish oil, curcumin, turmeric) or cause sedation (5HTP, tryptophane, valerian root) are more likely to help.
7. **Topical herbal supplements** are especially useful for pain that is close to the surface such as the arms and legs rather than the neck and the low back. Health food store supplements include Boswellia

Cream (an Indian herb with anti-inflammatory action) and DMSO (a wood solvent that dissolves the skin oils allowing rapid penetration, increased circulation and decreased pain). Often I recommend Boswellia Cream followed by DMSO (on clean skin).

8. **Topical prescription anti-inflammatory and neuroleptic medications** are now available in cream form at most compounding pharmacies. These are safe and at times effective. A common prescription is tetracaine and ibuprofen.
9. **Spinal adjustments** as performed by chiropractors, osteopaths and some physical therapists often decrease pain. Some people notice relief sooner than others and find it worth pursuing for several sessions if needed. It should be considered in most chronic pain conditions.
10. **Acupuncture** is the use of very delicate, fine needles. It is certainly one of the oldest tools for pain relief in the world. A growing number of studies verify its use for a number of pain sites especially the low back and neck. It is more helpful in use with electrical stimulation, moxibustion (a heated herb) and cupping.
11. **Biofeedback** is the use of relaxation training to relieve pain. It draws upon a very old method that uses the mind to bring the body into a calm state. Because there are many types of relaxation exercises from which to choose, the main goal is to find one that works consistently and then use it 1-10 times per day. The simplest method is to recall experiences in nature associated with comfort, contentment and vitality.
12. **Affirmations** are a focused form of mental healing energy. When combined with an active image of well-being it can invoke a laser-like effect on the source of the problem and accelerate recovery. The greatest effect occurs when a connection is made with the higher self, its basic design for health and wholeness. This is the main source of healing energy. When there is a cooperative relationship with the inner spirit healing is happening. One example is "I am healthy and well in every way for myself and each of those I meet this day."

13. **Counseling** is an essential part of chronic pain treatment. During our 12-day sessions we scheduled 2-3 counseling appointments per day. Resolving old issues is complicated and challenging. However the energy released with genuine expressions of forgiveness and insight is reassuring and healing at a deep level, aligning the emotional and physical bodies to a higher level of serenity, wholeness and healing.
14. **Laying-on-of-hands healing should be considered.** Some individuals have a special skill of normalizing pain conditions. Even if positive results are only temporary there is an increased confidence that healing is possible.

Chapter 8

Sources of Energy are Everywhere

Energy is a gift of life we often do not appreciate until there is less. "Youth is wasted on the young," George Bernard Shaw told us about a hundred years ago. But it is an ancient problem. We do not appreciate vibrant health and vigor until it is diminished due to illness, injury or aging. Fortunately there are many ways to increase energy and health no matter when or why the loss occurs, as long as we are willing to learn the lessons on the way.

We need energy to wake up, prepare for the day, perform the work to be done and take full advantage of the opportunities before us. The more energy we have the more eager we will be to plan the day and fill it with what we have to offer. It is also quite apparent that there are many different kinds of energy from gross and raw to subtle and sublime. The quality of energy is often more important than the quantity of it.

Fatigue is a common symptom of most acute disease, chronic disease and aging itself. There was certainly no reference to fatigue as a disease in my medical training, and I suspect it is very unlikely or even considered in any current medical training program. Even as a symptom it is largely unnoticed even though most people consider it a major quality of high-level wellness.

Many illnesses increase the demand of physical energy. Acute disease, whether from the flu or pain, often drops the energy level to some degree. As we recover it returns. At times what seems like a minor ailment is more severe and becomes chronic with one of the results being a continuing lack of usual energy. There are many causes of chronic fatigue, the most common being viral syndromes, mononucleosis, IBS, chronic pain, and depression. However there is also a condition called chronic fatigue syndrome that is a separate disease with specific characteristics. The required elements to diagnose it emphasize at least 50% less energy than usual for at least six months, no other diagnosable cause of fatigue and worsening symptoms with physical exertion.

Hormone levels decrease as we age and the result in lower energy. The most commonly recognized endocrine illness with fatigue is hypothyroidism, although it should be low adrenal function. In my experience adrenal gland deficiency occurs earlier and more frequently. Menopause and andropause, male menopause, are also common causes of fatigue. Each of these is associated with multiple hormone deficiencies and dysfunctions. Nerve hormone deficiency should also be in this category as well as a wide range of macronutrient (like insufficient protein) and micronutrient depletion (like magnesium and Coenzyme Q10). Most major mood disorders frequently result in energy loss and mental sluggishness.

The first goal should always be to diagnose the problem as well as possible. Most of the time a diagnosis can be made with proper history taking, physical examination and testing. Often a review of the sequence of events leading to the first sign of disease indicates the physical cause. With the usual symptoms of a sore throat, fever and fatigue, a viral infection can be assumed to be the triggering event. This is true for mononucleosis and also most viral fatigue syndromes, including influenza, IBS and certain kinds of arthritis. An accident or injury can also initiate a chronic condition such as pain, fibromyalgia and depression, all of which are often accompanied by fatigue. Emotional distress, fear and anger may result in anxiety, depression and fatigue effects. Stressful work relationships are also a major source of physical and emotional disruption and fatigue.

A Woman With Chronic Fatigue

A woman in her early 40s found herself having to return to work. Her two children were grown, educated and on their own. Her relationship with her husband was good but he lost his job in an unfortunate and unexpected way. She decided to return to elementary teaching and had no trouble finding a position in a school near her home. However she had to begin college classes to regain state teaching certification. The classes required that she spend her weekends attending and studying for up to two years for completion. The classes were not that difficult for her but the time required became exhausting. She had to establish new class work outlines for the children she was teaching and on the weekends study the course work for recertification.

After several months she came down with a flu-like syndrome. She pursued the usual remedies and eventually saw her family doctor. There was no detectable major illness, but she did not recover. The energy did not return. The cough and cold symptoms resolved but the fatigue remained. She continued her very busy schedule but remained tired all the time. She sought alternative treatments that helped to some degree, and she slowly recovered over several years.

The physical cause was a viral flu syndrome. The precipitating factor was the depleting stress of overexertion in a middle-aged woman. The immune system needs a reliable, consistent amount of physical energy to perform adequate maintenance and regeneration. Excessive physical and mental exertion with insufficient recuperative rest depletes the immune's protective capacity. What is usually a minor though annoying flu syndrome may become a post viral chronic fatigue condition.

Testing And Diagnosing Fatigue

A review of the history and an examination will often lead to an accurate diagnosis. Diagnosis and treatment are often aided by laboratory testing, including the usual chemistry panels but also, ideally, new innovative tests. The chemistry panel will show several items related to physical energy factors such as hemoglobin (for anemia), protein (for diet insufficiency), blood sugar (for hypoglycemia), iron (anemia), salt (for mineral depletion), and liver and kidney panels (hepatitis, fatty liver and aging kidney).

Many other tests can be ordered from a community laboratory related to a fatigue assessment. These would include vitamin B12, folic acid (B9), Vitamin D 25 and many hormones.

All labs do a thyroid panel. Ideally this panel includes free T3, free T4, TSH, thyroid antibody panel and reverse T3. The conventional test for screening thyroid dysfunction is the TSH test. It is thyroid stimulating hormone secreted from the pituitary gland which monitors thyroid function. TSH decreases when over-stimulated and increases when under-stimulated, such as with most hypothyroid conditions. As I describe in Chapter 6, basing diagnosis on TSH alone may not be a valid reflection of thyroid function.

The adrenal gland function is essential to assess fatigue conditions. It is commonly tested by an AM Cortisol level that is rarely helpful because it is at the end of a complicated series of many adrenal hormones. The DHEA Sulfate test is more likely to be an indicator of adrenal function because it is near the beginning of the adrenal cascade and reveals mild to severe depletion much earlier than cortisol levels. The gold standard test for hypoadrenalism is the ACTH stimulation test that is cumbersome and costly, though it is necessary at times.

Immune testing may reveal causes of low energy. It is commonly performed with the CBC (complete blood count). These are only gross quantitative tests, not functional tests and thus less helpful than assumed. The WBC count is the gross number of white blood cells in a microscopic space. Ninety per cent of the time it is in the low end of the spectrum in my patients because the immune system is not activated and fighting a major infection. Even in those with chronic mono or other viral syndrome the count is at the lower end.

There are tests that measure other aspects of the immune system when assessing fatigue conditions. The natural killer cell count has been shown to have correlation to the severity of a chronic immune deficiency syndrome, often associated with chronic fatigue. The immune cell complex includes helper and suppressor cell counts. It is usually done to monitor HIV infections, although it can be used for other immune deficiency syndromes.

The anti-nuclear antibody test (ANA) is a common test to screen for autoimmune disease. Borderline and low normal does not mean serious autoimmunity, however it hints at immune involvement. The higher scores with this test are of concern and are associated with diseases like rheumatoid arthritis and lupus erythematosis that are fortunately uncommon.

Antiviral antibody tests are used to diagnose mono, Epstein-Barr (EBV), cytomegalo virus (CMV) and herpes virus (HPV 1-6, A and B). These have some value, especially for acute viral syndromes to identify a recent virus. However, they are not necessary for treatment purposes although helpful in identifying a causative agent. Lyme disease and HIV screening are also necessary for severe, chronic fatigue syndrome assessment.

Fatigue lab assessment should often include women's and men's hormone function. Estrogen, progesterone and testosterone are all energizing hormones and need to be in optimal ranges for healthy vitality. Community labs can do these routinely. More complete testing, such as 24-hour urine specimens may be needed for a thorough view of function. For men, and at times women, the testosterone test ordered usually should be free and total levels. The free testosterone is unbound to protein. It is the active component of testosterone and therefore may be a more reliable indicator of true function.

A general rule of thumb is to evaluate these test results by looking for out of range values. I believe the ideal range is usually the upper half of normal for most of these tests, exceptions being the TSH and reverse T3, which should be in the lower half.

Growth hormone may also be worth assessing. GH levels fluctuate throughout the day and therefore we usually use IGF-1 (insulin-like growth factor 1) tests to assess this function.

Neurotransmitter function is a relatively new way to evaluate fatigue conditions. One method to assess it is by 24-hour urine testing. A spot urine test is more likely to be helpful although requiring optimal amounts of the protein precursors to be accurate. Although these tests were designed for rare hyperadrenal syndromes, they may provide indications for underproduction or depletion of these vital energizing nerve hormones. Anti-depressant medications do not affect these levels but 5HTP and tyrosine supplements do. These amino acids are direct precursors to serotonin and dopamine in the kidneys that is the source of urine for testing.

Other tests that may be of value include those for major vitamins, minerals and other chemicals. The vitamins to test are A, B1, B2, B3, B5, B6, B9, B12, C, D-25, and E. The minerals are magnesium, calcium, chromium, zinc, iodine, iron, sodium, potassium and chloride. The amino acids are essential and conditionally essential ones. The fatty acids are omega 3, 6, 7, 9 and saturated fats. Also worth testing at times are organic acids and anti-oxidants such as co-enzyme Q10 and alpha lipoic acid. One or more of these micronutrients may be important by causing a bottleneck deficiency which can influence many chemical reactions downstream causing noticeable functional effects of chronic illness and fatigue. A few cutting edge labs do comprehensive testing of these items such as Genova in North Carolina.

Psychological testing should be considered in most chronic disease including severe fatigue. This is a sensitive issue for many with chronic fatigue because the medical field discounted the diagnosis of it as a medical problem for many years. Those with prominent fatigue symptoms were diagnosed with primarily psychological conditions, not physical. This perspective is slowly changing and prominent investigators are leading the way.

Assessing the mood and mind is necessary as they often play a major role. Simple quick tests are now available for depression and the current state of happiness or lack thereof. At the pain clinic we measured patients with the Minnesota Multiphasic Personality Inventory (MMPI). We also asked what was an average amount of depression between 0 and 100, with 100 estimated to be the worst, depression to the point of not wanting to live anymore, 50% is half that and 10% a mild amount. Although very subjective it provides a comparison basis that is helpful with follow-up assessments.

It is quite apparent that most people with debilitating chronic disease have depression to some degree. At the pain clinic we found that most people had stressful events happen in life that were accompanied by sadness, guilt and anger. These often accumulated over time and led to serious difficulties affecting self-expression, self-identity and major relationships. Effective counseling can help re-establish healthy functioning and restore a full energy state.

Energy Medical Treatment

Medications can be very helpful to increase energy. My preference is to start with lifestyle changes as these are more likely to lead to greater healing over time. However, are many medications that should be considered. The categories of medication include thyroid, adrenal, estrogen, progesterone, testosterone, psycho-stimulant, sedating, antidepressant, and mood modifying.

The thyroid gland should be carefully assessed and treatment rendered. The art of thyroid treatment requires optimizing the medication options and supplements that boost thyroid function. Observing the response and repeat testing are often needed for best results. Pig thyroid or synthetic bio-identical versions of it provide T3 (tri-iodothyronine), and T4 (tetra-iodothyronine). T4 is the medication used by most physicians because studies showed that it is a bit more reliable in restoring TSH values to normal. However studies that take into account how patients feel in terms of well-being generally prefer whole thyroid. T3 is the active ingredient of thyroid hormone function; it works only the day it is taken, whereas T4 must build up over 6 weeks for optimal tissue saturation and effectiveness.

Adrenal gland prescription medication is in the form of cortisone. Prednisone is the most prevalent form, although hydrocortisone is bio identical, and may be safer. There are safe uses of cortisone when given in modest amounts for the purpose of optimizing adrenal function. When over the counter supplements do not work well enough prescription cortisone should be tried.

There are many kinds of estrogen and progesterone treatment. A thorough evaluation of symptoms and hormone status is necessary. Benefits and risks need to be considered carefully because of the fear of cancer in many. Although generally much safer than harmful, experimenting with various doses and combinations may be necessary.

Testosterone has value in both aging men and women. Although increased energy is the most likely value from testosterone, there are many other benefits. Increasing muscle strength is one of them, especially in those who exercise. In addition many notice increased cognitive function, concentration and memory. In some, the mood is also improved. A few will notice aggressiveness and impulsiveness. Other adverse effects include hypertension, acne, developing facial hair and loss of scalp hair. These are uncommon, especially with low doses but may occur.

Psycho-stimulants do help many, but not all. They are worth a trial. There are many types to choose from especially among the amphetamines. Adverse effects are due to overstimulation and are dose-related. Those who are prone to drug abuse or underweight should not use them. After being used more than a few months they must be withdrawn slowly, never abruptly.

Sedating medications primarily aid with sleep but can also modify general anxiety. Most people with fatigue do not sleep well and certainly do no awaken fully rested. There are many supplemental options and mental exercises that can be learned to treat these symptoms. Medication has a role, especially in those with major sleep disruption problems. If sedation is needed for anxiety during the day regular counseling and relaxation training appointments should also be undertaken.

Antidepressants often increase energy. They work by increasing the nerve hormone levels at the site of nerve connections. Nerve endings do not touch like wires that run our lights and appliances. The gap from one nerve ending to the next is connected by nerve hormone release. Antidepressants bridge this gap by enhancing the neurotransmitter contact. They do not increase the supply but improve nerve-to-nerve transmission. There are three main categories of anti-depressants: SSRIs, SNRIs and dopaminergic. If necessary each of the main categories should be tried for maximum benefit. Adverse effects occur infrequently but depend on individual propensity. They include anxiety, restlessness, less emotion, decreased sexual drive and performance and weight gain.

Mood modifiers are medications that generally have a calming effect. They are light to moderately sedating and so are especially helpful in anxiety states that include difficult sleep disorders and chronic pain. They have few adverse effects especially in the lower doses. They do not generally increase energy other than to modify certain conditions that improve the sense of well-being.

Energy Supplement Suggestions

There are a wide range of supplements that increase energy and decrease fatigue. The main groups of supplements are hormones, hormone precursors, herbs, vitamins, minerals and injectable supplements.

In general, over the counter adrenal hormone products are the most potent supplement stimulators of energy. The adrenal gland is the most commonly used. These are usually taken from New Zealand beef that have no reported cases of mad cow disease, and they are range fed. The adrenal glands are processed and prepared in capsule and liquid form. They are available alone or in combination with other glandular products but are more potent when taken alone. The capsules come in variable amounts and are usually taken following breakfast or lunch. If taken too late in the day or by an overly sensitive individual, they may interfere with sleep.

The most common adverse effect of adrenal gland capsules is heartburn that is less likely when taken after food. The liquid form is more potent and unlikely to cause intestinal symptoms especially when held in the mouth for at least 20 seconds before swallowing. Effects are generally noticed within 1-2 hours and work only the day taken. They do not build up over time. This is a reliable form of treatment for fatigue and helpful to many.

DHEA is the most common hormone secreted by the adrenals and has been the focus of a great deal of research. Books have been written about it. The medical field has not embraced it as a useful treatment, and many are more concerned for its adverse effects than its benefits. My review of the literature and experience with its use over 20 years indicates that it is very safe and often helpful, especially in those with abnormally low blood levels. It has been shown to improve the health of every major system of the body all of which have receptors for its functions. The muscles, bones, immune, cardiovascular and cerebrospinal systems all improve with its activities. The mood and memory have been shown to perform better as well.

DHEA is in the androgen category of adrenal hormones, which means that it has similar effects as testosterone. It converts to testosterone in approximately 70% of women, but less than 30% of men. 7-Keto DHEA is less likely to convert to testosterone or other adrenal hormones and in my experience is not as effective.

The adverse effects are not common with recommended doses of DHEA, although a few individuals are sensitive to even small amounts. In woman under the age of 50, acne lesions may occur in a few sites. In women over 50, there is a small chance of increased facial hair and loss of scalp hair. In men, there is a slight chance of increased PSA values, but otherwise it is very unlikely to produce other adverse effects. Levels are monitored by follow-up blood tests.

Two supplements are found in large amounts in the adrenal gland, vitamin C and B5. Therefore vitamin C is recommended in 1000mg amounts and B5 500mg/day. Licorice root has also been found to delay the breakdown of adrenal hormones as they pass through the liver. It can raise the blood pressure modestly so must be watched closely in those with hypertension.

The thyroid gland has building block ingredients necessary for production. These may optimize function of the gland as well. Iodine is the major mineral in the thyroid hormone; modest amounts can be helpful, excess amounts can inhibit secretion. Tyrosine is the amino acid building block; it is safe and well tolerated; 500-1000mg/day is recommended although it should not be taken without 5HTP, 50-100mg/day (10% of the tyrosine dose). Selenium and zinc may also improve thyroid function.

All the B vitamins increase energy by playing a role in many chemical reactions, especially protein synthesis. Blood tests can be done to measure levels. Again, upper levels of normal may be most beneficial. In general, a common recommendation is 100mg/day. Unfortunately, such a B complex may not be enough for all the Bs. Very few B complex products or multivitamins have more than modest amounts of B12 and folic acid. Some people need higher amounts. Instead of the usual 100mcg of B12 found in most B complex preparations, many benefit more from 1-5000mcg/day, and methyl B12 may be more effective than cyanocobolamine B12. Folic acid also has many benefits especially as a complement to anti-depressant medication. High amounts may also increase the energy level by optimizing neurotransmitter supply; 5-methyl folate is the most functional form and best amounts range from 1-7.5mg/day.

The mitochondria are the energy factories of the cell. Every cell has hundreds to thousands of these factories the purpose of which is to produce ATP, adenosine tri-phosphate. This is the fertilizer of all chemical cell reactions of the body. Two supplements play a major role in the production of ATP, Coenzyme Q10 (CoQ10) and NADH (nicotine adenine dinucleotide hydrochloride). Both have been used for several years to increase energy level. Much more research has been done on CoQ10. Although discovered in the U.S., Japanese scientists studied its use vigorously in those with heart disease. They found that it aids many with serious heart disease to recover faster and prevent recurring and progressive disease. It is also often recommended for fatigue conditions. CoQ10 blood levels are now readily available to monitor optimal amounts.

Helpful CoQ10 amounts vary widely from 30-300mg/day. A new form of CoQ10, ubiquinol, has greater potency, absorption and effectiveness. It is very safe. I cannot recall any patient of mine with trouble taking it.

NADH is the first of 3 steps in the final production of ATP. It is also very safe though less potent than CoQ10. Nonetheless it should be part of a comprehensive supplement program for overcoming fatigue. 5-10mg/meal is an optimal dose. Several products and programs have been developed to increase mitochondrial function. I am not aware of specific studies that verify their effectiveness. The rationale for their use is real, and the benefit may be worth trying. The few patients I have seen who tried these did not have problems taking them but also did not report major benefits.

Many herbs and homeopathic remedies are recommended for fatigue conditions. I am not aware of a consistent response with any one of these although others report they do. Ginseng and Ashwaganda are two of the most commonly tried.

Injectable supplements have an added effect in many people. B12 has a long history of use in physicians' offices. I often recommend 1-2mg/

injection, 1-2X/week for an initial trial. Traditionally B12 is used as an injection for treating pernicious anemia. For this condition, injections are recommended as 1mg/month. However many individuals, especially as they age, do not assimilate optimal amounts. Blood tests will often show low normal levels although below normal is not common.

A popular injection is a combination of B vitamins: B1, B3, B6, B12 and adrenal gland. At times these are more effective than taken as oral tablets.

Another common injection is the Meyers cocktail. Named after a physician on the faculty of John's Hopkins, he began these injections in the 1940s. Alan Gaby M.D. was practicing medicine in Baltimore and began to have patients of Dr. Meyers requesting these injections. Various modifications have been made but the basic formula is similar. The ingredients are B vitamins (1,3,5,6, and12), minerals (magnesium, calcium, zinc, selenium and multi-trace), vitamin C and marcaine, a long acting form of novocaine. These are commonly very relaxing, acting within minutes, and often enhance sleep the night of the injection. An energizing effect is noticed several hours to a day later.

Gamma globulin is a human immune protein product that is also energizing. It is medically indicated in immunodeficiency conditions that also include chronic fatigue syndrome (CFS). It has a history of use for travelers abroad to prevent infections. I have patients with CFS who receive it every three weeks to add energy. I also use it for those with non-CFS fatigue and those with frequent infections. It is very safe.

Nerve hormone replacement should be considered for everyone with low energy. These supplements usually use the amino acids tyrosine, 5HTP and cysteine. When taken to optimal amounts they can increase neurotransmitter function and subsequent excellent energy levels. This approach requires several tablets/meal but adverse effects are unlikely and results are quite favorable. A thorough discussion of these is available at neuroresearch. com.

Lifestyle Suggestions for Exuberant Energy

How we live largely determines the quality of energy of body, emotions and mind. Our habits of nutrition, exercise and activity establish much of the vitality of the body.

High quality protein, fat and carbohydrates help ensure macronutrient needs. These are usually met by lean meats, preferably fish and fowl, raw and cooked vegetables and whole fruit. Most people should avoid red meats, dairy (except yogurt), breads, pasta and most desserts. Range-fed food and organic produce are generally healthier with good amounts of protein and minerals. Water remains the best fluid and 6-8 glasses/day is recommended. Alcohol, salt and caffeine should be taken in only modest amounts.

Optimal exercise adds energy and strength for most people with mild to moderate fatigue. Severe fatigue prohibits much exercise. However most can do at least some stretching and cardio exercise and feel better when doing it regularly. Just walking 30 minutes/day meets minimum levels for a healthier exercised body providing sufficient circulation stimulation for multi-organ function. Outdoor exercise, especially gardening, also increases exposure to the sun and air, both of which aid the body in gross and subtle ways. For some people with fatigue, exercise is the treatment of choice and by itself restores most vitality.

The places we spend most of our time has an effect on the body's vitality. Some houses, offices and work sites are chemical or fungal factories, though only rarely a serious problem unless recently renovated. Noisy neighbors and streets can be a difficult distraction that must be addressed. Loud, smoke-filled sites are also energy depleting. On the other hand there are many areas and buildings that are refreshing and renewing. These include places of worship, healing centers, museums, gardens and many places in nature.

The emotional atmosphere of work relationships impacts the presence of quality energy. Intense work schedules can deplete some people quickly, although frustration, unfairness, pettiness and criticalness are far more debilitating. Marcial Losada developed the Losada scale that is used to evaluate the psychological tone and energy quality present in the work environment. It measures the extent to which the work environment may be affecting the health of its workers for better or worse.

The health of a company is determined by the number of positive to negative statements made by officials and staff of the company. The ideal ratio is 5 to 10 positives to each negative. Less than 3 to 1 is an indicator the company is not healthy and may not even survive very long. Over 10 may indicate excessive optimism to the point of unreality.

Our family and friends also create an atmosphere of healthy and unhealthy energy. The number of compliments and supporting statements versus critical statements affects our emotional body that supports the physical. The major relationships we have reflect the kind of person we are. These correspond to the energies of goodwill or dysfunction that go with them. At times it is necessary to move beyond the relationships and moods we have to establish healthier ones that we need. Kindness, civility and cheerfulness are often energizing and healing, and the basis on which to form new relationships and maintain old ones.

It is important to recognize that stimulating the mood and mind awakens them to greater alertness and energy. These subtler energies have a positive effect on our behavior. A personal program of enjoying nature, music, and art is often fulfilling. Such activities stimulate the creative elements within us. Reflective reading, meditation and church or temple activities may also contribute to the inner need for inspiration and creative activities. Similarly, hobbies, special interests and study groups may infuse the wellspring from which we draw our interest in living as well. Enthusiasm and curiosity are healing stimuli for the mood and mind.

The main lifestyle change to make is to choose the highest focus of intention. Setting forth the best use of time for a typical day can begin the process. Such a review is aided by considering the ideal use of the five senses, feelings, thoughts and intentions each of which can be a source of energy. This is not a small task but very worth the effort. The more we dedicate ourselves to our highest possible aspirations the more we tap into larger supplies of energy. The higher we reach the more we uplift, heal and renew ourselves.

Dedication to a noble cause draws forth a steady stream of energy that vitalizes the entire system. Unfortunately many of us are dedicated to satisfying our urges for comfort, pleasure, and protection. These have their place but need to serve higher goals. Most of us know what is most important and what we cherish but do not give them enough effort to dominate our lifestyle. These may include our children, a special talent or a cherished cause.

A cherished cause can be an excellent use of energy. Many individuals continue attending AA groups to maintain sobriety. Some continue the group meetings to support those in greater need than themselves. Other go further by becoming a sponsor or new group leader. These dedicated efforts draw forth the energy from the higher nature. Attuning to its agenda for us sends forth energy that is cleansing, nurturing, healing and uplifting to the rest of who we are.

A special talent in art, music, teaching, writing, counseling, a profession or common job done well can fill the need to have purpose. Any task or commitment to fulfill an obligation or care for a loved one in distress or with disease can be a cause. With dedication and persistence we draw forth power and energy that helps to ensure health and wholeness.

Nature's Laws of Energy

The parable of the talents by the Christ embodies the principle of the right use of energy. When the owner of an estate decided to take an extended leave he called his three main workers. Each had a different level of responsibility and therefore was given a different wage bonus. When he returned at a later time he requested their services and asked what they had done with the amount received. When the first two indicated they had invested and increased the earnings by tenfold he was delighted and took them back into his employment. The third one who had been given the least amount buried his gift to protect it out of fear of loss. When the master returned and heard what he had done with his money, he took back the amount given and told him to leave his estate, and not to return.

In our modern ways of working and interacting with compensation we receive, this treatment sounds outrageous if not illegal. The principle however, is that what we bury does not grow. What we do not use withers. The presence of the physical money is real but the value of it diminishes over time. What is not used generally loses value. Our higher talents and expressions also lose value if not used. Faith, hope and strength must be used to grow. So, too, our higher aspirations must be re-awakened regularly to increase their capacity to breathe in the vital air of new life. Our indwelling spirit has more to offer us when it has a platform of enthusiasm and optimism to work through.

Based on well-recognized principles there are at least three major laws of energy. The first one is that "we reap what we sow." Seeds we plant in our hearts and minds determine the type of feelings and thoughts we call forth. Fear attracts more fear. Anger grows with greater expression. Giving up leads to greater depression. And the reverse works as well, so that goodwill leads to good luck, friendship attracts generous helping hands when we need support and honesty leads to trust and opportunity.

I saw a patient recently who was in the area to visit his daughter. He had a minor medical condition requiring attention. During our discussion I happened to notice that he worked for the government and asked in what way, to which he said the state department. I related my only contact with a former ambassador to a European country and how delighted I was with the visit, hearing insights about the people, about their history and the complexities of issues he faced. It turned out he was on the staff of that embassy when that ambassador was there. He said that this ambassador was great to work with, friendly and skilled at confronting crises. Most of all he said that the ambassador respected all those he met. It was not surprising that he was also the most favored ambassador the country had ever had from the United States. He sowed goodwill, genuine interest and respect. In turn he was regarded highly, trusted and supported.

The second law is that energy is multi-dimensional. In other words we can draw upon higher levels if we seek them out. Relationships are multi-dimensional because of the feelings and thoughts that radiate through them. Forgiveness, tolerance and gentleness are more energizing than resentment, intolerance and harshness. Clever and thoughtful humor is more energizing and regenerating than crude, rude and critical humor. Honesty and integrity bring greater trust and cooperation with others than do blaming and complaining.

"To get a new project off the ground go to the busiest person in the group" is a common saying. People who are active in many ways are more able to make decisions quickly, involve people easily and generate new ideas creatively. Being plugged into the spirit of the task at hand often helps the ideas of the mind to connect to the attitudes most needed and the actions that best express them. When health is failing or a chronic condition becomes depressing, it is necessary to re-ignite ourselves with a new vision of why it is important to be well. Returning to the health we had is often less than what we are can do. The old reasons to be well may have led to the current limits and so a new mission must be found. These in turn increase our energy and interest in living.

I recall a patient who attended the Meadowlark Retreat Center. When I first saw her she was using two canes to walk, moving slowly. She had rheumatoid arthritis that had progressed to a major degree. During her stay she learned more about diet, exercise and the sequence of events that led to her condition. By the end of her stay she was better but still encumbered. Several months later she returned to the center and was a totally different person, walking without canes and exuding enthusiasm. Wondering about what happened and hoping we may have contributed to her new well being I asked what caused the major change in health and energy. Although there were various factors it became clear that the main difference was a new relationship of love and delight. A wonderful new companion and all that it brings can affect everything about us including a healing of the body. Relationships are often multi-dimensional, energizing us in heart, mind and body.

The third law of energy is that more is given to those who use well what they have. As we learn the language of a new skill, challenge, crisis or relationship and move toward mastery of it, we increase our freedom of opportunity for learning and growing. The more people with whom we interact the more we learn about how life unfolds. The more skills we develop the more creative sparks come alive. As we choose wisely on what we ponder and express the better choices we find in friends and fulfilling activities.

The most important key to health and happiness is social connections. The more we have the healthier we are physically and emotionally. There is less disease and when it happens we heal faster. There is less depression and anxiety because we have more folks to remind us about the seasons of life, the bounty of life and the cycle of good that is bound to return. The more people with whom we associate the more opportunities to express who we are and see the results. We gain from the appreciation and learning how to heal.

The opposite occurs as well. The more we criticize and complain the more we limit our options to improve our circumstances. The more we withdraw from those around us the more we miss from other's experiences of what works and what doesn't. The more we blame others for our losses or illnesses the more we miss learning the skills we need to heal ourselves.

Learning how to use the laws of energy helps us plug into the universal energy supply. Like the law of gravity we learn how to use laws of life to propel us forward, to heal our ailments and enhance our well-being. As we learn how energy flows to those who use it well we can propel ourselves to greater success as well. As we become a channel of its benefits to others we become a vital part of the expanding energy of love, wisdom and joy. This is how we mobilize our healing power.

Express Loving Kindness and Understanding

Chapter 9

Transform Stress to Stimulate Healing

Stress is part of living. We come into a very imperfect world and learn quickly that we do not simply get what we want and what we think we need. Life is not for the meek and mild. It is harsh and very incomplete.. The solution is to realize that we are here to make it better. We are called to not only survive but also thrive. Life is filled with sources of abundance that we are meant to harvest. Stressors in our lives are the growth points of opportunity that challenge us to discover the strengths we have, how to express them and what we have to contribute. Finding how we can serve the greater whole leads us to the skills we need to learn. The more skills of living we develop the more stress we can handle.

Stress is a reaction of concern to wants, needs and events that happen. Maslow describes a hierarchy of needs that begins with physical survival, safety and basic comforts. Stress includes a wide range of emoting fears, doubts and worries and also enjoyments, kindnesses and caring. As we refine our feelings, there is greater freedom to be curious, explore our interactions, and develop greater knowledge of healthy living. The highest needs involve the energy and guidance of the higher self to find meaning and purpose in all that we do. We are designed to mobilize the higher needs to uplift the lower ones.

Emotional stress raises the risk of death. A recent study reported in the *British Medical Journal* surveyed over 68,000 adults as part of England's National Health Survey from 1994 to 2004. The more depression and anxiety a person reported having, the more likely they were to die. People with mild distress were 29% more likely to die of heart disease or stroke than people who reported no distress. Mild distress didn't seem to raise the risk for cancer. People with moderate levels of distress were 43% more likely to die of any cause. And people with high levels of distress were 94% more likely to die during the study than people with no distress.

Stressors are the individually defined triggers that lead to a stress reaction. They include a wide range of physical and psychological challenges to meet the vast array of our physical and emotional appetites. The Eastern sages focused much of their wisdom on the *I Ching*, the book of change, which is the simplest description of a stressor. Change in our daily routine, our diet, the weather, and relationships trigger stress in varying degrees. In turn these changes set in motion continuous swirling emotional energies of the present intermingling with the past, constantly changing who we are.

Over 50 years ago Drs. Holmes, M.D. and Rahe Ph.D., began to study the effects of events as stressors of change. They compiled common events and then tested them rigorously, resulting in a way to quantify the effect they have on most people. The stressors they studied in descending order of importance included death of spouse, divorce, marital separation, personal injury, retirement, gain of new family member, change in financial state, line of work, living conditions, residence, recreation, social activities, eating habits and vacation. They identified as many positive as negative changes. The more change in a short period of time the greater likelihood and severity of injury and illness.

They found that even accidents and injuries occur more frequently in those with more stress in their lives. They conducted a study in the Navy on a shipload of sailors. Over the first 3 months at sea, they found that those who became ill or had an accident were the ones with the highest stress score. They performed a test on the University of Washington college football team showing that the high stress players were more likely to incur serious injuries.

It didn't matter whether they were starting players, the better ones, or those on offense or defense. During the study Dr. Holmes began to feel guilty by allowing the high scorers to continue to play.

Especially intriguing is their finding that we all need a certain degree of stress. There is an optimal amount of stress necessary to challenge us to be active enough. We each have a range within which we function best. Too much stress may overwhelm us and not enough is boring and depressing. Unfortunately, the common response to stress is to get over it as soon as possible and learn how to avoid it. The healthy approach is to use stress as an opportunity to add new attitudes of the heart and attributes of the mind.

The Ways That Stress Lead to Illness

The physiology of stress is simply the body's response to stressful events. This is basically a survival instinct to protect itself. Learning the principles of how the body responds to stress helps us appreciate its complexity and give us clues to its regenerative capacities.

Much stress is triggered by an outer event, a physical or emotional interaction outside ourselves. The brain is the main center through which stress is transmitted to the rest of the body. Generally we need to decide something is stressful before it is experienced as such. Choice is involved although most choices are a result of habit patterns based on earlier choices made. Often much stress is felt without much thought or choice because of our habit patterns and instincts of reaction.

The brain responds to stressors in two major pathways: the nervous system and the endocrine system. The nervous system sends signals to the sympathetic apparatus that alerts its entire network, the intensity of which varies with the urgency of concern. From the brain the energy of stress passes to the spine, with sympathetic nerve chains on either side of the spine. In turn, these send impulses to descending, smaller branches that spread to the rest of the entire body. The sympathetic system wakes up the body to warn it and prepare it for impending stress. The parasympathetic system that primarily influences digestion, assimilation, elimination and sleep, is diminished along with its capacity to rest and renew the body.

Specific neurotransmitters are the complex chemical messenger agents connecting one nerve to another, which activate the major organs of the body. The nerves stimulate the heart to increase its strength and frequency of each heartbeat. These in turn increase breathing of the lungs to provide the basic energy of oxygen to meet the demands of greater cellular activity. With increased blood flow the muscles are filled with multiple nutrients and more capable of full motion and mobility.

While the nerve network, cardiovascular and muscular systems are stimulated under stress, several other organs are diminished via the parasympathetic system. Like an intricate electrical grid, energy is allocated by need for urgent action. The organs of digestion, assimilation and elimination are lessened. The chemical energy demand of the stomach, intestines and urinary tract are diminished. This shift is safe, natural and healthy for short term uses of acute stress. However, long term, persistent stress will harm the body if these functions remain lessened.

The second major pathway of spreading the stress response throughout the body is the endocrine system. This is also a complex interacting cascade of intricate chemical hormones with receptor openings on every cell of the body. Within the brain is the pituitary gland, the master control gland with hormones that regulate each of the other hormone centers. The first one to increase is ACTH, adrenocorticotropic hormone, which stimulates the adrenal glands to greater activity. These hormones in turn increase energy by the dual action of tearing down old cells (cortisone, cortisol) and building new ones (DHEA, testosterone). The adrenaline-related hormones have an immediate effect while other hormones have a more delayed action.

It is a marvelous wonder of creation to consider how the body works. In the short term these system responses fully awaken the body for action and mobility. The senses are activated providing the astute input necessary. A wide array of options becomes available to avert danger or pursue the prey.

If sustained for more than brief periods of time, the systems become depleted and disease develops. Organ breakdown depends on age, intensity of stress, duration of stress, inherent genetic weaknesses and lack of regenerative capacities. Early signs of strain include hypertension, headaches, fatigue or pain in any system. There are a wide variety of medical conditions that can ensue, in part predictable by prior stress experiences and family predispositions.

Hormone system deterioration also occurs in similar patterns. Initially there is an increase in hormone output that may register a high or high normal level detected by laboratory assessment. Over time sustained stress will eventually lead to depletion and under function of gland activity. Each gland has its own indications of excess and deficiency, manifested by symptoms, physical signs and lab testing.

Illnesses From Stress

There is no one illness that is definitely, consistently due to stress. Causes of disease are multiple including diet, injury, environment, genetic predisposition and a range of other factors. However most illness can be worsened, become more recurrent and less likely to heal as a result of undue stress.

Heart attacks can be precipitated by stress. Many studies now support the triggering role of stress in heart attacks. When I was in medical training on the cardiology rotation, I undertook my own brief survey. As part of the initial history taking of those with confirmed heart attack, I included a question about stress. I interviewed ten consecutive patients diagnosed with a heart attack. Eight readily identified major stress within the last three months. The wife of one man pulled me aside a few days after his admission to ask if a certain event qualified as stress. A few months before his heart attack, he was at work driving a heavy tractor. A close friend was walking nearby, following him in his tractor, chatting as they walked. He reminded his friend to not walk too near the tractor since it could be dangerous, especially on a recently rained side of a hill. His friend continued walking nearby until the tractor began to slide down the hill sideways, trapping his friend between the tractor and another heavy machine. His friend became paralyzed from the waist down, and her husband began to feel terrible for several weeks just prior to his admission to the hospital. She asked whether this qualified as major stress. Of course it did, big time.

One of the classic studies on stress and hypertension was undertaken by Herb Benson. He studied the role of stress and hypertension in young men, the most vulnerable group for high-risk heart and stroke disease. He focused on the treatment of hypertension with relaxation. He found that the relaxed state lessened heart rate, respiration rate and blood pressure. Even those with the worse prognosis of hypertension, young men in their 20s, could normalize blood pressure with twice per day relaxation sessions. As long as they did this, they did not need medications to normalize blood pressure. He reported his findings in *The Relaxation Response.*

Sleep dysfunction is often a result of accumulating stress. A 72-year-old woman came to the office with insomnia. She was going to sleep at 9:30 PM and awakening at 3:30 AM but was unable to return to sleep. With a full day's schedule she was increasingly exhausted. She had a history of other medical problems but not insomnia until two weeks prior to her visit. She was requesting herbal suggestions to help her sleep.

When asked what has been going on in her life she finally admitted to a major concern over a close friend who was dying of cancer. A few weeks before the insomnia started he began to require full nursing care. However, his money for the extensive care was limited. He had a large fund but it was not available for two years. She was the executor of his estate and didn't know how to help him. I suggested that she set up an appointment with a bank loan officer to make arrangements until the money was available which led to a resolution and better sleep. This obvious solution had not been considered but was associated with great relief and return to normal sleep.

Addressing the source of the problem is usually more beneficial than lessening the symptom. The most common sense solution is often not considered under stress. Although medication and supplements may be helpful and temporarily necessary, healing the source of conflict is even more desirable.

One Thursday afternoon a patient of mine began to have mid-back pain. It rapidly worsened to the point of tears and inability to work. I encouraged her to go home to rest, use ice and take Advil. The next day she returned to work feeling somewhat better and able to work. She had gone to the emergency room where they ordered a CT scan of the abdomen and low back, which was normal. On further questioning she related the stress that was current in her life. She worked full time, raised two young children, played softball two nights a week (plus tournaments on the weekends) and attended night school. In a few weeks is test time. She has a great deal of study work to do but was not caught up in her preparation for the tests. After our discussion, she restructured her study schedule, her softball time and family support for the children. Lessening the stress decreased the pain.

A young man in his fifties was concerned about a new rash that he never had before. He thought it might be shingles but wasn't sure. It was on one side of the body, a small patch of blisters and itching. These are characteristics of herpes zoster, known as shingles. He was wondering if medication should be started immediately, even before he could be seen for an appointment. He was not in major discomfort and preferred not to use medications and so I recommended to wait until his appointment the next day.

When I examined him it was clear that he had a mild case of shingles. We talked about the various aspects of it including the cause and timing of it. I shared with him that it is commonly a result of physical and possibly emotional stress and that usually there is physical strain that precedes the appearance of skin lesions by two to ten days. He then related an event that occurred about a week earlier with his dog. While he works his young dog is home alone but allowed to use the yard. A few days before the rash he came home to find the dog having played with and damaged a few new plants in pots. He scolded the dog and repaired the plants. On this particular night he came home after a 12-hour work day and found several plants torn apart and strewn around the yard. Furious with his dog he became very angry and chased the dog around the yard trying to properly punish it and finally teach it the lesson of leaving the plants alone.

The strain of chasing the dog in a tired, angry state set him up for undue stress. Most likely the back muscles were overworked and triggered a reaction. The anger caused an alarm reaction that provided the energy to chase the dog but also depleted him more, as well as the immune system's ability to maintain normal stability. The virus of shingles, latent in the spinal cord, had more food from worn out cells dying slightly faster than usual, and they multiplied rapidly into an outbreak. For him there was a high degree of physical and emotional stress. Fortunately he realized his error, the over-reaction, and took steps to heal and prevent it from happening again.

Common Ills Can Be Triggered by Stress

As a family physician I see many people with the common cold. Even though we know it is caused by the cold virus, usually from the rhino virus family, I often advise people that the onset can be triggered by stress. I have seen enough studies and patients to be convinced of the connection. Only recently did I experience it myself. I rarely get sick. There is an occasional flu and cold but I can't remember missing a day's work in over 35 years. I may have lightened a day or cancelled an event but never missed a whole day.

It was with special interest I noticed events unfold that triggered a typical cold virus response. I was warned the night before by my wife that a letter had arrived in the mail but that I probably shouldn't look at it until the morning. I am a morning person, awaking early, full of energy and eager for the day. In the evening, I unwind and retire early, usually asleep by 10-10:30 PM. In the morning there was a brief open time for a few minutes. I opened the letter and noticed that it was from Medicare, the insurer for about 20% of my patients. They were conducting an audit of several patients, asking for copies of the progress notes for one particular day for each patient. We had been warned a few years before that they would be surveying some physicians. In fact, I was surveyed a year before for the extended type of appointment, meaning a longer period of time spent. However, this survey was for the shorter visits, the typical visit that most doctors use to record an appointment, probably representing 75% of the daily load.

The shocking thing to me was the request for records of the regular patient visit to the office. I had been quite aware of the need to record a proper number of items of the visit for the history and the exam for several years. Now they were auditing the charts to see if this was being done. My problem, as with many doctors, was having legible notes. They were legible to me but not to most others I'm sure. So, I would have to type these up myself and submit them. That was not so much the problem as the realization that other insurance companies like Blue Cross and Blue Shield would also likely follow Medicare and begin to audit chart notes as well.

While I was seeing patients that day, in my mind I extended Medicare's request to the other insurers and the future began to look bleak. There would be an initial investment cost of no small amount and, even worse, a learning curve of several hundred hours, meaning several months of less than fulltime work to set up the new system. The fear began to spread rapidly. The only solution I could fathom was to bite the bullet and develop electronic health records (EHR).

While my mind is reeling with the new set of obligations I felt a sinus strain and began to feel a nasal drip. This was the initial sign to me of the on-set of a cold virus. The congestion began and the nose began to run. However, in the middle of this I remembered the local hospital's offer to join the staff in developing EHR. I called to set up an appointment to have a review of the system. It was easily arranged.

The next day was Saturday, and, fortunately we had already scheduled a computer expert to visit the house. While he was working with our son on his computer I remembered a draft of a new progress sheet I had written several months before in response to the first audit. It was a detailed paper record of what the computer program would provide, i.e. circling items of the history and exam on paper instead of with a mouse for a computer graph. My wife offered to do what she could to advance our ideas on the draft form and then the consultant proceeded to complete a usable form.

It was almost exhilarating to see it printed out. It would require a full size page per visit compared to the usual page providing space for 5-10 visits. Nonetheless it would work and not require electronic health record learning time and money. Within minutes there was a definite sense of relief and the dripping nose stopped. I had not experienced something so dramatic with my body before. Sinus congestion continued of a very minor nature but the cold did not progress the way they usually do, i.e. major drainage, cough, bronchitis and continuous congestion for several days. The sudden onset and rapid cessation was a new experience, confirming what I had seen in others and dramatically demonstrating what is possible with a new strong direction. Resolving the stress abated the usual progression of disease.

How to Treat Stress Once It Has Begun

Acute stress is frightening but treatable. The heartbeat is fast, the breathing cannot keep up with the apprehension, and panic is everywhere. It is like a fire alarm bell going off right next to you. The sky is falling and you can't get away. This state usually requires medication. A primary care physician should always be available or someone to call who can and will act on your behalf. If not accessible within a short period of time, I recommend going to an urgent care center or the emergency room. They know how to treat severe acute distress efficiently.

Most people need a calming agent immediately or else suffer for several hours. There are several medications available by prescription and most of them work well within 30 minutes. The only over-the- counter medications that provide a sedating effect are the antihistamines like Benadryl or Contact.

There are alternative remedies that help some people in early stages of acute distress. These would include Rescue Remedy, a Bach flower essence combination found in most health food stores. At times people have a pre-arranged herb or other supplement that has been shown to work such as theanine, 5 hydorxytryptamine, lithium orotate or sublingual magnesium. These have a relaxing effect within minutes to an hour that is sufficient in many. They may be especially useful if taken on a regular or as needed basis to prevent mild to moderate stress from accelerating.

The old remedies of a long hot shower or bath have some value. An even better idea is calling a friend, mentor or counselor if available and capable of handling such an event.

At times the best action to take is leaving the setting in which the stress is happening. If you are in a restaurant and the inner alarm goes off, excusing yourself for a few minutes may make a big difference. Even going to the bathroom to get away should be considered. Getting outside and inhaling fresh air may be helpful. The amount of oxygen outdoors is greater than indoors; at times a crowded room will deplete the energy content of the air dramatically and inhibit a healthy stress response.

Ideally there is a process available within ourself to work it through. Most of us need time to review the significance of the stress we feel. With time to think it through we can identify the trigger and the built-in fear, frustration or anger associated with it. As we observe the reaction, we may be able to identify the beliefs behind it and ways to change it. This is usually not simple or easy but with concerted effort, insight and patience, new patterns can be created and new, healthier beliefs chosen.

If severe acute distress is a common occurrence, a list of options should be set up for ready use, including medication, people to call and a medical facility to visit.

How to Prevent Severe Stress

Everyone experiences stress of variable intensities from time to time. Only rarely do people have a panic attack requiring urgent attention. Most people can benefit from learning about causes of stress, how it works and how to prevent it from causing disease. There are no simple strategies to managing major stress because of the complexity of who we are and the many different parts of our inner nature. But there are many simple steps which can contribute to creating a sense of calmness. Over time we can develop a subtle energy shield of serenity that protects us from major stress.

The initial goal is to have a healthy body. We are usually not dealing with acute physical trauma but inner, emotional conflicts. Nonetheless, having a healthy body will minimize the experience of acute stress because it is has greater resilience. Exercising regularly keeps the body in good condition and helps us be more attentive to overdoing. However, we also need to eat well and get sufficient rest. Lapses in any of these healthy lifestyle routines increase the risk for the experience of physical stress and detriments from it.

Knowing how the body relaxes can be very reassuring. After working at the Pain Clinic with Dr. Shealy, I became very impressed with the value of relaxation skills. People with severe, chronic, post-operative pain conditions can learn how to markedly diminish and prevent pain with relaxation training. The medical literature is now filled with studies documenting its value for a wide range of illnesses including various stress conditions. Developing the skill of relaxing and doing it on a regular basis prevents stress in the body by increasing the tolerance for it. Relaxing regularly also increases the sensitivity to foresee which stressors may become serious and how to confront them effectively.

Simple techniques for relaxing begin with setting aside the time to relax. Preferably this would be done nearly the same time each day and performed regularly. The body anticipates its routines and actually begins the process of relaxing before the time arrives. It can become quite automatic, like putting on our clothes, eating a meal or driving a car.

Getting into a comfortable position and breathing deeply triggers a relaxation response. Calling to mind a common experience of being relaxed connects our nervous system to a soothing calmness and quietness. Using a mental exercise for relaxing the body can easily deepen the experience. When done regularly we generally have a more relaxed body most of the time. We also become more sensitive to our own common stressors and the ability to develop skills that manage them better.

Most of the strategy for preventing stress occurs within our heart and mind. One of the most stressful times in my medical training was preparing for my internship year. This was the first year in which we made decisions ourselves. We had a more trained physician available to us but were expected to make quick assessments and treatment decisions. I had a dream in which I was presenting myself to an official of some kind. He was seated at a desk reviewing my situation and said, "Tell me your 50 best characteristics." After telling him something I don't recall, he said "You should be going to Cornell."

This was a very reassuring dream. I was raised in North Dakota, and although excelling in high school and college I did not consider myself in the Ivy League category. I took the dream seriously and wrote out 50 positive qualities of myself. I was not used to doing this but eventually completed the task. The results were a definite elevation of confidence and courage. I did perform well during my training years.

Listing your strengths and skills will work. Studies have been done by Martin Seligman, Ph.D., and others identifying the value of signature strengths work. They have found that designating the top three strengths and looking for ways to express them each day has a tremendous impact on health and well-being. Those who do so for only one week notice an improved measurable mood up to six months later. I suspect the primary benefit is from continuing to practice the exercise after the first week because we find it valuable and effective. The reason this exercise works is that it increases our self-esteem and self-image when practiced regularly providing an insulation layer of self-reliance and tolerance to stress.

Reviewing peak events transforms stress into resilience. Peak events evoke courage, optimism and a sense of discovery, along with a willingness to set aside old ways of thinking for what is new and potentially better. Peak events are often a mixture of many loose ends coming together into a single theme or focus. They are worth careful study and exploration so that we extract all the good possible. They can include many types of music, art, literature and theater. These expand our oases of well-being and quick access to them. These are the ways to overcome the more common tendency to dissect the traumas and tragedies and re-live the pain instead of the wisdom gained.

The Ultimate Cause of Stress

The primary cause of stress is the presence of life within us. It is designed to promote growth and learning in our body, heart and mind. The mission of the higher self is to compel expression in whatever circumstance we find ourselves. It is like the Bible story of the mustard seed as a metaphor of heaven. The tiniest seed has the capacity to grow and expand its presence over a much larger area than its appearance seems to suggest. It must confront the weight of soil over its head, the boulders in the way, lack of moisture and competing plants for the nutrients available. The seeds of life within us continually respond to the opportunities that arise. These seeds include courage, commitment, insight, kindness, caring and cheerfulness. As circumstances arise and we become engaged in them, these seeds come to life to help us express our inner humanity and contribute to the larger life around us in spite of obstacles in the way.

The primary purpose of stress from within is to add our life to the greater whole in which we live. We are meant to be here and have our part to play in the larger drama of life. It has meaning and purpose. The more we contribute, the more we are filled with its life, strength, love and joy.

Skills for Enlightened Stress Management

1. A healthy diet that moderates stimulating substances like coffee, spices and sugar.
2. An exercise regimen that emphasizes heart action without exhaustion; e.g. an equivalent to walking three miles in 60 minutes.
3. Beginning the day with reasonable goals of action and accomplishment.
4. Requesting from within the strengths needed for the likely events and people of the day.
5. An active day of work or creative activity in office, home or elsewhere.
6. Confronting the challenges of the day with eagerness, confidence and courage.
7. Setting aside one to two break times of quiet reflection and relaxation for 10-20 minutes.
8. Including a little time for art, music, poetry and nature.
9. Ending the day with gratefulness for the best things that happened and all those who contributed to it.

Chapter 10

How to be Relaxed, Calm and Confident

Relaxation is what the body does naturally when not in use. It is a state of resting calmly and comfortably. There is minimal muscle action, slower heart rate and diminished breathing. Physically, relaxation is controlled by the parasympathetic nervous system, the part in charge of rest and sleep. During this state major organ function is quieted down while the digestive, elimination, immune and regenerative capacities are increased.

Psychologically, relaxation is a state of serenity that allows for a greater review of the current state of feeling and thought. During this state the energies of the most recent events and interactions are more apparent for observation, exploration and new direction.

The body knows how to relax well because it does so often. Every night we go in and out of sleep. During the night the body moves from light to deep to dream states of sleep, back and forth several times. During the day it also moves in and out of high alert to low alert cycles. Some suggest that these are roughly 90-minute intervals during the day.

Other than sleep at the end of the day, the most natural time to relax is after eating. There is no doubt that relaxation is easier after eating. The blood flow increases to the abdominal area to digest, assimilate and eliminate the foods taken. The blood flow decreases in the brain and muscles diminishing their function. The shift in circulation triggers a relaxation effect to slow us down to digest our food better. The warnings to not swim after eating are based on this significant shift of circulation. The body cannot empower major muscle action and the full digestive process at the same time. For this reason after lunch is an excellent time to encourage the body to relax itself and adjust to the energy changes of the foods we eat. It is also a good time to review and adjust the feelings and thoughts of the day.

Every physical activity has a natural cycle of relaxing after finishing its tasks. The body seeks to eliminate the chemical wastes that accumulate from physical activity and replenish the cells with fresh nutrients,. Both of these functions require a shift in circulation from the center of an organ to its surface, from the center of the body to the periphery, from the trunk and brain to the arms and legs. The shift in circulation is what causes a subtle but noticeable warmth and heaviness in the arms and legs. No one wakes up with cold hands and feet unless without sufficient cover.

Upon awaking is a good time to register how it feels to be relaxed. This memory can recreate the relaxed state. Early morning is also a good time to program healthy intentions and strengths for the day as well as reflect on the unfolding events to come. This is a good time to decide whether to emphasize enthusiasm, optimism, patience, persistence, calmness or confidence. These attributes minimize stress and enable relaxation during the events of the day.

Medical Conditions That Improve With Relaxation

During the time of relaxation, renewal and regeneration are increased. Relaxation improves most medical conditions especially to relieve excessive strain, stimulation, worry and concern. Although causes of most conditions are complex, excessive strain will worsen them while an optimally relaxed state will enhance healing. **Common diagnoses that respond to relaxation are pain, hypertension, asthma, anxiety, and insomnia.**

Any **muscle tension syndrome improves with relaxation intervals.** Acute and chronic pain respond readily to simple relaxation exercises, although lasting effects also require the cultivation of healthy moods. Elmer Green and associates at the Menninger Institute studied the healing effects of relaxation and biofeedback on migraine sufferers several years ago. Their research inspired other studies that also established relaxation training as a beneficial treatment approach for many conditions. As a result Dr. Shealy established the Pain and Health Rehabilitation Clinic, the most comprehensive outpatient pain treatment program at the time. When done effectively and consistently relaxation is often a very reliable treatment for chronic pain relief.

Hypertension is another common condition that responds to the relaxation effect. Herbert Benson M.D. studied and popularized this effect. He found that two 20 minutes sessions per day lowers blood pressure to normal levels. Initial studies were performed in people in their 20s when the diagnosis of hypertension has a lifetime prediction of medication use. He showed that this is not the case in those who are consistent in their use of relaxation intervals.

Hypertension is more prominent as we age. It is also complicated by family history, weight changes, medication use and a variety of other factors. It is a very frequent diagnosis that is treated almost exclusively by medications that in turn have a number of adverse effects. Relaxation training should be recommended to almost everyone with hypertension. It is safe, easy to learn, inexpensive and effective.

Other cardiovascular conditions may also respond to relaxation training. Various tachyarrythmias that may be felt as palpitations are often associated with increasing stress in personal and work environments. Most cardiac diagnoses are worsened by stress. A regular program of relaxation during the day may help prevent the effects of stress as well as diminish usual predictive trends of gradual worsening. Medication use should always be monitored by the physician, but patients should also request medication adjustment when there are signs of positive response to relaxation efforts.

Irritable bowel syndrome involves a wide range of chronic intestinal dysfunction conditions. The pain that often accompanies IBS is due to muscle spasm of the intestinal wall. This action is mediated by nerve impulses generated by inflammatory conditions. We can communicate with the nerves in the solar plexus during relaxation and minimize muscle action. Constipation is also commonly aggravated by increasing tension (this is one of the reasons it especially occurs when we travel.) Relaxation releases the accompanying tightness helping to re-establish natural peristaltic waves for a comfortable discharge of waste. Anyone who is toilet trained can learn how to relax and re-program healthy intestinal function.

The whole respiratory system is worsened with stress. During my medical training years I rotated with an allergist who was very dedicated to kids with asthma. He founded an asthma camp called Bronco Junction, built with a railroad theme. The kids stayed in railroad cars and, in times of need, could be transported to the clinic by a kid-sized train that ran from one end of the camp to the other. The summer I was there the alergist conducted a study of the benefits of relaxation on the occurrence and intensity of asthma attacks. The results clearly showed the value of teaching and encouraging twice-daily relaxing periods. We discovered that relaxation was very effective especially at the first awareness of an asthma attack. There were approximately half as many attacks in the relaxation-trained group compared to the non-trained group. In my medical experience, most adult respiratory conditions improve as well with even minimal suggestions to be calm and comfortable.

Sleep disorders often begin with major frustrations and anxieties. There are quite a variety of causes of sleep dysfunction especially associated with aging and hormone changes. However, relaxation training should be near the top of the treatment list of options. Relaxation is mainly a mental exercise that trains the body to focus on images and suggestions that shift the nervous system to a soothing, serene state. Insomnia disorders often result from excessive commands to worry, to act quickly, and to expect more to be done than is reasonable in a day's activities. These expressions awaken the sympathetic part of the nervous system creating a "red alert" so often and so intensely that the nervous system is unable to shift to the parasympathetic function in charge of rest and sleep. Relaxing memories and thoughts can reverse this process. More serious sleep conditions require attunement to the center of healing within, awakening the reservoir of forgiveness, devotion to the ideal and the pursuit of right priorities.

Anxiety experts and worry warriors are a more difficult group to relax. Mild forms respond quite readily to relaxation training. However, chronic, genetic and traumatic forms of anxiety require extensive training in not only relaxation but also depth insight work. Effective counseling can make major inroads in discovering the oasis of well-being that can become a center of self-confidence and comfort. Within each of us is a center of optimism, hope and joy. We just need to learn where to look. Most people with severe anxiety have become drunk on disappointments and have dug a deep hole in which they are surrounded only by what has gone wrong, how much they don't have and how little help is available to them. Part of the solution is a diligent effort to retrieve memories of success large and small. It is important to find reasons for gratefulness, and the goodwill of those around us. When these memories of real experiences are part of a relaxing period major positive changes do occur and most medical conditions improve.

The Physical Benefits of Calmness

The physical benefits of relaxation are multiple and affect every organ of the body. Essentially, relaxation helps to decrease the strain and increase the regeneration of the cells of each organ to full function. The systems that especially respond include the muscular, respiratory, cardiac, intestinal, nervous, cutaneous and endocrine.

In relaxation the muscles of the arms and legs decrease their demand for energy and are replenished with nutrients needed. Tightened muscles that relax allow for better delivery of nutrients and more efficient elimination of used chemicals such as lactic acid. Damage is repaired and new cells are more easily produced and maintained. Reserves are built back up for coming activities.

In the calm state the lungs and respiratory system slow down and the muscle bands around the breathing tubes loosen allowing greater flow of air. There is a more efficient extraction of oxygen from the air and more thorough release of carbon dioxide and other gas wastes. As oxygen is the single most vital substance needed every minute of every day, optimal lung function is essential for maximum health. With stress there is a tendency to hold our breath. With prolonged stress, we may develop a habit of inadequate breathing patterns and mild to moderate insufficiencies of this vital substance.

The heart begins to respond quickly to less activity. It is the most active muscle of the body and is designed for a certain number of beats per lifetime. Giving it a chance to restore and renew itself is of immense value for health and longevity. Conscious relaxation can lower the heart rate when needed as well as normalize irregular beating. Although instinctively it increases with worry and major concern, a calming confidence can also be learned to protect the heart.

When relaxed the abdomen is more able to function as the master chemist it is. As food is introduced to the stomach it responds quickly with hydrochloric acid to separate food particles into a pudding-like consistency. The pancreas behind the stomach produces many enzymes, complex proteins, that complete the process of digestion. The 20 feet of small intestines are in charge of assimilation, absorbing the nutrients so they can be distributed to all cells of the body in the simplest forms possible. The large intestine withdraws fluid and prepares the residue for elimination. The liver receives the nutrients absorbed and further processes them, neutralizing potential complications and preparing them for final use by the individual cells of the body. The kidneys filter the circulation, discharging the used byproduct and facilitating greater access to the nutrients needed. All of these organs of the abdomen function more fully in the relaxed state and are diminished in the very active and stressed state. Regular periods of inactivity allow them to function best.

During a rest time the nervous system builds up its supply of vital chemicals. The neurotransmitters found in the nerve endings do most of the work of responding to the five wonderful senses of sight, sound, taste, smell and touch. As they are replenished there is greater capacity for processing feelings, thoughts and interactions of the day enabling us to respond, remember, plan and prepare for what is next. Relaxation helps us maintain a refreshed nerve system coordination keeping us alert to our surroundings. It allows us to be more able to communicate our needs and express the good we have to offer those with whom we interact.

The skin system also has its need for overcoming excessive stress and being relaxed. The cutaneous system not only protects us with an elaborate detection complex but also eliminates about 5% of the total body waste. If the gastrointestinal system falters or becomes dysfunctional, the skin may have a greater burden and can become overwhelmed in trying to process more than it is designed to do. Stress can lead to skin eruptions in susceptible individuals and relaxation can treat and prevent this from happening.

The endocrine system of the thyroid, adrenal and many other organs also function best when given intervals of relaxation. Strain will increase their functions for short periods of time, but if prolonged will result in depletion, fatigability and accelerated aging changes. These are the organs that can generate immense energy chemicals in a crisis but require restoration time for repletion and recovery.

Psychological Healing Benefits of Relaxation

The benefits of relaxation are more than physical. A quiet time allows a chance to reassess emotional expressions, to process what has occurred and reevaluate interactions of the day. Relaxation provides the preliminary step to calmness, healing insight and meditation.

Calmness is the energy of creative quiet time. It is a time for renewal and regeneration, a time for detaching from the usual interactions and reactions. It is especially a chance to access a higher perspective that shows us how the dots are connected and how the piece of the puzzle we are working on fits into the larger landscape of life. As we reach for greater meaning we find greater calmness and confidence to do the tasks before us and enjoy them more.

Calmness can lead to insight. When relaxed and calm it is natural to review the most recent interactions with others and the emotional reactions to them. There is a ping-pong effect with every contact. It is especially apparent with expressions of severe anxiety, deep depression and outbursts of anger. However much less noticeable feelings of others affect us as well. The instinct of sympathy is strong so that our subconscious responds like a mirror that is alive. The sad story we hear triggers a sad story we've been through that is of a similar nature. This is especially common when a major event occurs such as an earthquake, flooding or violence. We must learn to observe our pattern of response. As we see what must be done to change patterns of reacting we can repair our reflexive emotional involvement. In the process of redoing how we react we also prevent the worst from happening and eventually learn how to choose healing energies more quickly.

Calmness gives us the chance to become an expert, super alert observer. The fictional expert criminal investigator Sherlock Holmes is known for his careful detection of the small but real details that eventually draws forth the culprit. As we become calm we increase the chance to review our reactions, however small, to the most recent feeling energies expressed and experienced. If these are of irritability, impatience, and mounting frustration we will be drained of the energy of goodwill and gentleness. We need to reach for our inner reservoir of patience and poise. As we sense the prickliness of blaming and complaining, we need to reach for forgiveness and tolerance. Distress and despair may respond best to our sense of hope and faith in our ability to grow and learn. Weariness and weakness may be uplifted by calling forth our innate capacities for resolve and resilience.

The more we claim our inner resources of calmness the more we can heal ourselves. The more we heal the most recent scrapes and dents of our emotional body, the more capable we become to go back in time and heal the deeper wounds. In the relaxed, calm state we are more able to observe our inner world, call forth the healing resources available and send them where needed. In these ways we mobilize our healing power.

Where Relaxation Fails

Physical conditions need to be diagnosed before they can be treated. Most symptoms are not signs of serious disease but many of them indicate that an effort should be made to explore further. Seeing a physician, having an examination and appropriate testing is recommended to identify potentially serious problems. If you have concerns that are becoming chronic, consult with someone who knows more. This is never a guarantee that all has been done. In the process of looking further we set in motion our own inner alert mechanism for evaluating what is happening, and we awaken ways to find resources of healing.

Serious problems need more than relaxation. Lives are saved every day by emergency and urgent care medicine. Medications relieve pain and suffering on a vast scale. Surgeons perform necessary procedures that restore health, comfort and greater function. We should consult these experts when needed and at least listen to suggestions of those who may know more than ourselves about current concerns.

Most major worries, anger and depression require far more than relaxing exercises. Serious psychological conditions require a concerted effort of self-assessment, identification and expression of the strengths within. Professional counseling is often helpful although finding the best counselor may mean trying a few. In counseling the emphasis should be on reviewing the peak events and virtues unfolding as well as focusing on unresolved conflicts. Long standing habits of avoiding responsibility, self-pity and resentment of others do not heal quickly.

Medications may be needed. Although my preference is to try a healthy lifestyle of nutrition, exercise and healthy activities, these may not be sufficient. There are numerous supplements, herbs and homeopathic remedies that may complement efforts to be well and should be pursued. However, medications are more concentrated and are more likely to bring about positive changes quickly when necessary.

Far beyond relaxation and calmness is our inner capacity for insight, inner guidance and common sense. By setting aside time for reflection on the current concerns, we can often access a healthier perspective and reasonable expectations. Many times we simply do not know enough about ourselves and the complexity of the issues involved. With patience and persistence we can slowly gain knowledge and wisdom and the confidence needed to rise above what we now see as obstacles to our life.

Simple Steps to Relaxation and Regeneration

1. **Take the time you need**. Setting aside the same time each day is very helpful. The body begins to anticipate the approaching time to relax and actually begins the process as the time approaches. 10-20 minutes is sufficient for most.
2. **Choose the right place**. It contributes to the body's receptiveness to suggestions for relaxing. Feng Shui is the art of creating harmony of furniture and decorative objects in a house. This is also helpful to add harmony to our innate needs to be comfortably relaxed.
3. **A comfortable position begins the process.** With only a little experimenting this is easy to do. Uncrossed arms and legs and loose clothing are a good idea. Reclining during the day that leads to sleep may not be best.
4. **Close the eyes and notice the immediate effect on the body**. This is an important step that begins the relaxing process. A major source of stimulation is diminished quickly. Pay attention to the letting go of residual muscle tension that is set in motion.
5. **Learn one relaxing exercise that works well.** There are many that include breath observation, muscle tightening, or pleasant memory retrieval. One of my favorites is to address each part of the body slowly and methodically, noticing first whether there is any strain, then asking that to stop, followed by specific instruction to relax. For example: "Relax forehead, relax." Appreciate the response received whether noticed or not, and ask that it spread throughout the surrounding area especially to the next area chosen. After starting with the forehead move to the eyes, face, jaws, tongue, neck, shoulders, arms, chest, abdomen, back, legs and feet.
6. **Focus on the body breathing itself.** Feel for the gentle wave of relaxation that flows across the body with each breath out. It is like a pebble thrown into a pond that sends ripples to the end of the pond. With each breath out, there is a ripple of relaxation that flows down the arms, into the hands and out of the fingertips and thumbs. It flows

from the chest, through the abdomen, down the legs and out the ends of the toes, with each breath out. Slowly the body sinks deeper and deeper into the chair or couch or bed with each exhalation.

7. **Choose words that are relaxing**. To relax even further you may use the words quietly to yourself, on breathing in, "I am," and on breathing out, "Relaxed." Do all that you can to relax deeply and completely. Sinking deeper and deeper with each breath out.
8. **Choose a memory of a place in nature that is relaxing and renewing.** It doesn't have to be perfect, just a pleasant memory. It could be a place spent on vacation or a walk alone in some lovely scene or setting. Listen for the quiet sounds and the energy of the air. In the mind's eye find a comfortable place to recline and do so. In the mind's eye close the eyes and continue saying the words "I am…relaxed."

When done regularly the body learns how to relax for you. As this skill is learned look for the benefits that occur over time. This evidence then becomes a more compelling reason to relax regularly one to two times per day especially during more difficult times. Even during stressful times you will find the body relaxing at least a little during the designated habit time developed.

The relaxed state is an excellent time to review recent events and interactions. This is the time to reflect on sources of strength within and the virtues you most seek to find. This is the time to rehearse how you would like to use the energies most needed and practice how to express them better. Invoke a strength needed and imagine expressing it. Expressing calmness heals anxieties and worries. Expressing courage heals fears and doubts. Expressing cheerfulness heals somberness and sadness. Expressing respect and reverence heals anger. These are the ways we draw upon the center of peace within, the peace that passes understanding, that leads to healing body, heart and mind. This is how we mobilize our healing power.

Chapter 11

Relationships Generate Growth and Self-renewal

Relationships are a means whereby we experience the personal world of people around us. Relationships with others connect us to our reasons for being and the wide array of expressions and enjoyments they bring.

The family unit is the springboard to relationships with others. Though often less than ideal, mother, father, brothers, sisters and the extended family are the sources of our early interactions. For better and for worse, these become the models for how to take care of ourselves, how to express ourselves, how to heal, how to relate to others and our world view. For those without family members, prominent people, real and imagined, teachers, neighbors, friends and sometimes foes become role models for relationships.

As we mature from youth to childhood we begin to interact with others in school and our neighborhood. We slowly extend ourselves into our community and discover a wide range of relationships. In the school setting we relate to students of our own age and a few who are younger and older. We learn how to relate to teachers and develop our experiences with authority. Eventually we learn how to relate to co-workers and supervisors. In time we may become a parent or role model to family members and others in our community largely based on what we have learned from these early relationships. This is the cycle of life with widely variable amounts of learning occurring at each of its stages.

The key lesson in relationships is love and its many attributes of gratitude, forgiveness, tolerance, self sacrifice and loyalty. All of these are awakened by emphasizing shared goals and shared responsibilities.

Extend Gratitude Often

Gratitude is one of the easiest ways we learn about love. Even our dogs and cats express gratitude often. Being thankful for the efforts extended our way helps increase the energy of graciousness and generosity. Words of praise are just the beginning of healthy appreciation. Demonstrating it is the real thing with acts of kindness, support and help where needed.

Recent studies confirm the healing effects of gratitude. In F*lourish* Martin Seligman discusses several studies on gratitude. One study asked participants to identify one person who has meant a great deal and to whom not enough appreciation has been expressed. They were directed to write a letter describing the major ways they were helped by this individual. After writing the letter they were encouraged to arrange a meeting with the important person in their life without alerting the person as to why. At the meeting, they were to read the letter and pursue the interaction that followed. Those who did this exercise felt a better measurable mood of happiness for on the average of one month.

One patient of mine wrote to an old friend who is now her daughter's godfather. They dated for a while until she was compelled to break it off due to his heavy alcohol use. Soon thereafter he was involved in a life changing motorcycle accident. He became wheelchair-bound and in chronic pain. Their relationship diminished to the point of little contact for several years. When asked to write a letter to someone she had not thanked enough she chose him. She highlighted the goodness and strength he had shown her. He was deeply moved by her gratitude. She heard how much he regretted his treatment of her for many years. The experience of sharing the letter with him and discussing the memories revived their friendship and is benefiting all of them.

A series of other experiments have developed into what is called the "three gifts exercise." Participants are asked to write down three good things and why they happened during the day. The items don't have to be dramatic or earthshaking, simply enjoyable or worthwhile. These may include interacting with people we care for, an interesting bit of news, the triggering of a fond memory, an insight, a funny story, listening to pleasant music or the warmth of the sun on a cool day. Those who do this every night for one week have a better mood for at least three months. The extended benefit is probably due to the fact that once you start a healing habit you see and feel the value of it. Consciously and subconsciously people choose to continue it because of the positive effect it has.

Gratitude is a celebration of the good in our lives. It draws us closer to sources of delight with our family and friends, nature, music, art and the higher part of ourselves. Even small acknowledgments increase our positive psychic zone, damping down the fears and worries at least temporarily. The more we pursue the skill of appreciating life the closer we commune with the higher elements of it and the source from which it comes.

One of my fondest memories of gratitude occurred during medical training. During my residency in Family Medicine I received a call from a resident in Pediatrics. She was from the Philippines, very kind and considerate although we were not particularly close. She called to say that this was her Thanksgiving Day and she was calling a few people to thank them for being in her life. It was the middle of May and a lovely gesture.

Gratitude dispels negative moods of distress and depression. There are many ways we isolate ourselves from others and dwell too much in our own world. As a result we are more susceptible to fears, worries and low self-esteem. Gratitude connects us to the lives of others, their goodwill and generosity. It also broadens the link to our own inner guidance and sense of value. These empower us and extend the good we have to offer others.

The healing effect of gratitude is in the action of it. Thinking about those to whom you are grateful helps lift yourself up. Feeling deeply appreciative definitely penetrates our layers of sadness and isolation. But actually expressing it expands our positive self to the deeper layers and shadow side of ourselves. "Thank you" helps but even more do acts of kindness, attending to small ways to increase comfort and diminish stress. Asking for how to help and initiating efforts to do what you know would help are genuine acts of gratitude.

The main source of gratitude must always be ourselves. No one knows the good we do, the right intentions we carry and the efforts we make. Too often we depend on others to recognize who we are and the ways we contribute to those around us. It is helpful and at times necessary to expect and require some degree of recognition and appreciation. Some people need to be reminded how we help them. However, a regular dose of self-acknowledgement will prevent the sense that we are not appreciated enough and be enough to satisfy us most of the time.

Gratitude is not always a positive expression. When done for self-centered reasons it is deceptive. The simplest example is a child wanting a favor, gift or special food from mom or dad, and behaves in a solicitous manner to obtain it. The more complicated versions develop as we become smarter and more discrete. One of the most effusive messages of gratitude came from a patient of mine who was grateful for receiving a pain relieving medication. His attitude changed as I necessarily, slowly withdrew the medication and had to refer him to another physician for further care. At that point he became quite angry and convinced I did not like him. The outer expression of thankfulness is easy to perform. It is important for us to learn to recognize the inner presence of genuine praise from what is not, especially if there are reasons to be suspicious of the motive behind it.

The obstacles to gratitude are many. Like physical exercise on muscles a generous heart requires many acts of giving. Lack of the use of gratitude is probably the most common obstacle to its expression. More serious obstacles include major agitation, anger and arrogance. Each of these forms of self-centeredness limits the ability to recognize the benefits and need to express gratitude.

The highest expression of gratitude is to the source of our being, the unseen though knowable life within. Each of us is connected to a source of life that is vitally interested and dedicated to our life and all our relationships. It helps guide us to heal from trauma, accidents and illnesses. It helps us make major life changes and develop important relationships. The source of our life deserves gratitude for what it has done over long periods of time from the obvious turmoil to the seemingly simple daily routines. Gratefulness helps us attune to the higher self's agenda as well as how to cooperate with it for our best growth and all those with whom we interact.

Forgiveness is the Re-set Button

Relationships grow with forgiveness. Forgiveness is a major gift of close relationships. Instinct helps us overlook minor conflicts but the real thing is necessary for the larger bumps in the road. Close friends and family will forgive readily. Most often it is not direct but indirect by not becoming a major focus of attention. The more healthy relationships we have the more likely forgiveness is readily available with some exceptions. However, serious violations of trust and loyalty will sometimes end relationships if not addressed quickly and completely.

To forgive quickly and deeply is a skill that requires serious consideration and continual effort to master. Fortunately much more is spoken and taught about forgiveness than there used to be. The simple words of sorrow and forgiveness are one thing while the sincere expression of them is something more. Genuine regret is a willingness to say "I'm sorry, that was stupid of me, please forgive me." It starts with a willingness to review what is said and done for the purpose of improving our expressions of goodwill to those around us.

Forgiving others starts with forgiving ourselves. Until we regret our own acts of rudeness and crudeness and accept the need to forgive ourselves, it is hard to extend forgiveness to others. Only as we forgive ourselves and learn to invoke the energy of forgiveness can we share it.

The need for forgiveness is enormous. Too many of us are too quick to blame and complain. Even many authorities set the wrong example by failing to admit wrongdoing and regret it. At times those around us do need to hear what they did that was annoying, neglectful and deceitful. Serious abuse must be recognized as soon as possible and challenged. We should always assess our own role in allowing or encouraging mistakes of judgment or expression. The harm we do to one another leads to major distress and disease that can continue for years and even decades. Unfairness, dishonesty and outright malice are present in too many. Although many of us are above criminal behavior most of us get angry, very worried and distressed too easily. Forgiveness is one of the ways these negative energies can be healed.

I remember a fit of frustration that led to an angry outburst to my young son. The expression on his face was so painful I felt it deeply for some time afterwards. We can't change the past but we can do our best to heal it. Simple genuine expressions of remorse begin the process quickly. Learning to use forgiveness often is an essential skill to healthy relationships.

I have patients who have been harmed by other physicians. It is not common but happens. Recently one patient was accidently given Hepatitis C by a faulty injection. She became very angry and afraid because she could not afford the new treatment that became available. Forgiveness may not become an option for some time although it is always available. Forgiveness is not for the other person but for ourselves so that we do not carry hatred, spite and loathing. These cause disease and pain physically and emotionally until healed.

Serious harm caused by others is not easy to forgive. Before forgiveness comes acceptance of the reality of what has occurred. Often over-reacting to insults or accusations of blame trigger emotional fear, frustration or anger and diminishes our awareness of what really happened. With acceptance comes a cooler review of who said what to whom and why. Gathering the facts is often very valuable because it helps us clarify the source of distress and the part of us inside that feels most threatened. The old adage of hunting applies here: "Aim small, miss small." The more we know our specific weakness and point of fear or anger the more we can respond with integrity and responsibility. Overshooting and over-reacting often amplify the problem instead of confronting it directly. We frequently see prominent people worsen their problem by not addressing it honestly and effectively. We often need to learn how not to do the same with our own issues.

Forgiveness is a way of loving ourselves and others. When we are to blame for certain problems we can mobilize the energy of forgiveness for ourself. It will help the healing to begin. All harm can be repaid, though patient and persistent efforts are necessary for serious blunders. Forgiving ourselves helps us set aside regrets, worries and mistakes of judgment. Forgiveness provides the chance to start over again, smarter and more sensitive than before. Forgiveness helps us rise above the conflict and disagreement to find the larger picture of which it is a part. Our relationships are opportunities to develop the art of forgiveness and slowly learn how to master its expression.

Tolerance Extends Our Boundaries

Tolerance is a companion of forgiveness. With friends we are tolerant but less so with others. However tolerance teaches us how to listen to and learn about new ideas, new ways of thinking and better ways of enjoying the life we have. Tolerance does not mean agreeing with something we oppose. It does not mean being kind when we should be critical or supporting something we don't understand.

Tolerance ensures the spirit of fairness in our relationships. It helps us be more broadminded and circumspect instead of too ready to decide what is right, what is wrong and how to correct misdirection. Tolerance helps us explore the many sides of complex circumstances and relationships. It is looking beyond the obvious differences of race, creed and country to the differences in temperament and reactiveness. Some are too readily responsive; others are stubbornly controlling; some are quietly intellectual and others are especially creative. Yet each type of perspective has its value and benefit in a relationship. It is up to us to learn how to relate to each type of approach, gain what we can and interact in productive ways.

Tolerance helps us to heal ourselves. As we are fair to ourselves with reasonable expectations we draw forth new opportunities to nurture our way through difficulties. As we are more patient and kind with ourselves we reduce the damage done from excess remorse and frustration. As we are gentle with ourselves we can heal the wounds that have been self-inflicted. As we heal ourselves we are more able to be a loving influence on those with whom we live and interact.

Tolerance increases our patience with ourselves and others. Tolerance means we are willing to think through what is being said or done until we learn more about it. We are willing to explore its significance. If it has value we can support it. If we gain insight about ourselves or others from what we hear and see, we can celebrate it and be grateful. Tolerance enables us to be more likely to learn from everything that happens around us.

Self-Sacrifice Deepens Our Bonds

Family and friends expand our world as we help each other. They provide us with many experiences, challenges and feedback we need to grow into our greater potential. Relationships require give and take, giving up what we would like that we can cooperate better. Choosing preferences over demands makes a difference in learning to live and work with others. In committed relationships there will be fluctuations over long periods of time. There are periods of days to weeks when more patience, support and sensitivity for the other is necessary. And at times when this is reciprocated. As long as the greater purposes of the relationship are honored and invoked regularly these periods will be opportunities for greater growth and mutual benefit. Balance is necessary but we must be sure to do our part.

The key to fulfilling relationships is sacrifice. The sacrifice of personal wants and wishes, comforts and preferences to the relationship makes room for a broader range of experiences. To sacrifice means to make sacred. Sacrificing self's interests increases the opportunity to look beyond personal needs and ways of feeling and thinking. Because we have limits to our physical existence in the physical plane, we need to let go of certain attachments to make room for new ones in heart and mind. The spirit of sacrifice enables us to do so.

Sacrifice does not diminish or belittle ourselves. It is not meant to allow abuse in any form. Unhealthy sacrifice may result from a desire to rely on someone else to make our decisions. If we enter a relationship for what we can get, for what can be easily gained and what makes our life more comfortable, we will be relinquishing our ability to grow and gain what we need for ourselves. The purpose of developing a relationship is to learn what each has to offer. This not always easy as one of my patients shares:

> "It was mid-December, and I had a routine appointment with Dr. Kwako. I felt so bad I considered canceling the appointment. I had agreed, after much pressure, to a month-long visit with my difficult ninety-one year old mother in Oklahoma over Christmas and the New Year. I felt simply miserable, dreading the trip itself, dreading Oklahoma and really dreading spending that much time with my mother. We have never gotten along very well, but as the only remaining sibling and as a daughter I felt I had a responsibility to go. To make things worse I felt really guilty for feeling the way I did. I was frazzled with Christmas activities and trip planning and my anxiety about the long stay with my mother was just adding to a big pile of misery.
>
> "So when Dr. Kwako asked me how things were with me, instead of my usual "fine," I told him just how miserable I was. He said 'Let's talk about this.' Wonderful words to hear, because very few people want to really talk about another person's misery!
>
> "First he told me I had absolutely no responsibility for my mother. I did not have to do anything about her I did not want to do. I was perfectly free to remain in Santa Barbara. This was shocking and I think I tried to argue, 'Aren't children supposed to be responsible for their aging parents?' No, I was not responsible for her. I was free to do as I wished.
>
> "He said some elderly people get selfish as they age and think only about themselves. They are not the same people we grew up with. I felt a big burden lift off my shoulders.
>
> "I almost canceled the trip. But for some time I've tried to do *the right thing* whenever I had a decision to make, finding it just makes life simpler. I decided that going to visit my mother was the right

thing to do. Believing I had a choice about it rather than a responsibility to do it made all the difference.

"I went on the trip. But the first time my mother started in on me about something I had done she didn't like, I could think much more clearly about how to handle this. I told her I wasn't used to living in an environment where people yelled and spoke harshly to one another and asked her to stop doing it. She looked amazed, she cried, we hugged each other, and she never did it again the rest of the visit. I call that a breakthrough."

Sacrifice can mean to end old ways of relating to the same person the same way and instead create a new connection that is more sacred and loving.

Loyalty Lengthens Relationships

One of the greatest gifts of family and friends is being able to rely on them especially during times of difficulty and major change. "Through thick and thin" is the common phrase that describes a close relationship. However being loyal is sometimes very difficult. Part of loyalty is truth-telling even if it risks the relationship. And sometimes loyalty is misleading attachment.

A close friend in high school became a primary grade teacher, head master of an open school and eventually author of three books. At one point he became engaged with a woman who did not seem like a good match for him emotionally or intellectually. I met her and spent some time with them. A few months later I was invited to their wedding. Upon hearing the news I was distressed because of my concern for him. After much consideration I decided to write him a letter explaining my view of his decision, essentially trying to discourage him from marrying her.

He proceeded with his plans and I attended the wedding. They seemed to be fine for several months until things began to break down. Eventually he divorced her, became depressed and was out of work for several years. He moved to another community, became a college teacher and met a woman who has become a wonderful wife and mother of their two children. And we continue to be in close contact. Our loyalty to each other has enriched us both over the years. It was not easy to confront him about such a huge decision but the right thing to do. He could easily have rejected me for many years to come but chose not to do so, his own spirit of loyalty to our relationship.

Loyalty is a character strength that binds people together. On the surface it is evident by the frequency of contact and enjoyable exchanges that occur. At the deeper levels it provides honesty, reassurance, forgiveness and commitment to help during difficult times.

In marriage loyalty strengthens the relationship so that it can weather the storms. And there are many storms in most relationships such as where to live, which car to buy, which friends to develop and how to cope with difficult family members and friends. The greatest joy and challenge is having and raising children. Loyalty is a force that expands and sustains all major relationships.

The spirit of loyalty is a glory to behold. A patient of mine recently heard about the death of her ex-husband. They divorced several years before due to his drug and alcohol addiction. He squandered money they did not have, was gone without explanation for lengthy periods of time and occasionally was emotionally abusive. He attended recovery programs but ended up in and out of jail.

After she found out about his demise she considered writing to his mother. She felt an urge to express heartfelt sympathy of some kind. Although she never had children herself she considered what it must be like to have a son die early from substance abuse. She asked my advice about what to say. I suggested that she write about the positive expressions and events he did contribute in their time together.

She proceeded to write his mother hoping it would be of some help. A few days later she received a response that was a profound statement of gratitude. His mother was desperate to hear something positive about her son. She was deeply moved to hear from her daughter-in-law with whom there had been little contact although no ill-will. My patient was very grateful to have made the effort to extend her concern. She had not realized it would have such an impact on his grieving mother. This is the spirit of loyalty from a woman to a mother-in-law and indirectly to her ex-husband when many others would have remained bitter or at least indifferent. Loyalty is a healing force of power when used well.

How to Develop Healthy Work Relationships

The work setting has a profound influence on our health and well-being. We spend the greatest alertness, strength and action to assigned tasks of the job. Fortunately for some it really is a mission of love and a worthwhile endeavor. For too many it is a reluctant task mainly to support our basic needs and those of our family. Unfortunately for others it is a trial of severe stress that is not only dull or boring but very burdensome.

One patient of mine recently reported a major change in her work relationship. For several years she has faithfully worked in a professional office as a trained assistant. Her employer was highly trained in his profession and demanded careful attention to detail. But he was also abusive, at times blaming her for circumstances beyond her control. He was easy to anger and frequently required schedule changes without notice or discussion. On one particular day a patient complained about the effects of a procedure in which she was involved. He became very angry, blamed her for the situation and then fired her. She was quite surprised because similar events of a worse nature had occurred without resulting in such a display of outrage or even threat of firing. She was deeply disappointed as she knew how much she had sacrificed to overlook his short temper and irrational behavior. She also needed the job to support herself.

She began to look elsewhere for work. Within a few weeks she was led to another professional in the same field of training. In the interview she relayed all that had happened with her previous employer. She was concerned that his professional loyalty might have excluded her from consideration. To the contrary he quickly reassured her that he was surprised she stayed as long as she did with such an employer. She was hired, has more benefits than ever before and, most of all, is treated with the respect she knows she deserves. She is also more aware of her own role in allowing the abuse that she suffered to occur.

Healthy work relationships can be the reward from patient, persistent efforts to do the best we can.

Relationship Karma

Karma is a beneficial balance in life. The essential meaning is encapsulated in the ancient phrase that we reap what we sow. It is a myth that karma is only getting your due of suffering. It is much more than being stuck with bad circumstances set in motion by bad decisions at some prior time. The reason we associate karma with difficulties, especially in relationships, is because we tend to emphasize the negative far more than the positive. Karma builds upon the unfolding growth and maturing of our character. It is more likely to emphasize the positive aspects of who we are in the relationships in which we find ourselves. Certain strengths are more likely to be active and self-restraint applied at the proper times.

Life has a wonderful way of balancing out what is missing. When I returned for a high school reunion it was wonderful to meet old friends. One couple was especially doing well. He was a good friend throughout grade school and she was a sweetheart near the end of high school. They are now both successful lawyers in the hometown. Her father died early in life and she was raised primarily by her mother. His father was gone most of the time and he did not have brothers or sisters. The two of them have two children and a wonderful family life, much more than each had when growing up. They found and created a family life that each did not have. The life force balance is at work in most of our lives if we look closely enough.

What we do not get for ourselves we may find for our children. A patient of mine was going through a difficult time. In asking more about her situation she was still quite aware of how much good was in her life. She and her husband each came from very difficult childhoods. Both families were very dysfunctional with excess alcohol and many other problems. They met each other when young and had two exceptional children. They did their best in raising them, supporting them whenever they could and helping them through challenging times. Their son did well in school and was accepted into Stanford. He completed his degree and now is very successful in business. Their daughter also has done well and was accepted at Princeton with a scholarship. What they did not get in their own lives they were able to provide for their children. This is far more often the case than not.

The instinct in most parents is to sacrifice for their children so that their lives are better than they had. Many accomplish it by providing a greater sense of support, sensitivity and stability to their children which increases their chance for a successful, enjoyable life.

Recovering from bad karma quickly is a skill worth developing. When I was working at Meadowlark Retreat Center I was struck by the story of a middle-aged woman. She told us that we are not always stuck with what happens to us. We were discussing difficult marriage relationships when she chimed in to tell us about her marriage. She said she knew it wasn't going to work on the day they were married. She decided that the only way to change the situation was to work her way through it. She decided to look for a woman that she knew was more compatible with her husband than she was. She arranged for them to meet and slowly spend more time together. She encouraged them to see each other at various gatherings and enjoy each other's company.

At the right time she expressed her desire for the relationship with him to end and for him to pursue the relationship with the woman he was already quite attracted to. They divorced and the other two were later married. It worked out that way smoothly and with no repercussions. She was thrilled and had no regrets, having prevented untold problems from her unhappy marriage. With insight and a clever creative effort we can be an agent of setting things right before they get off track.

Relationships Continue After We Die

Often relationships with family and friends are not perfect. Most assume that the time of death ends the opportunity to continue to enjoy and work on our major relationships. Many experiences suggest that this is simply not true.

A good friend was raised in part by a stepfather who was at best indifferent and at worst cold, critical and unhelpful especially in times of need. Never feeling very close she went through life wondering what little good he was to her. Recently she awakened during the night and felt her spirit apart from the body. It was an out-of-body experience. She felt herself go through the wall easily and found herself in a lovely setting where the light was bright and the atmosphere profoundly peaceful. Her stepfather appeared, greeting her warmly and saying how pleased he was that the family was doing well. He said that he was sorry he didn't treat her better but that he didn't know how. He wanted her to know that he felt differently now and was doing what he could to help.

After seeing him she felt a resolution in the relationship. It made sense to her to not hold resentments of any kind against him and that the lack of relationship she had with him was not due to her own wrongdoing. This was powerfully healing to her.

Making peace with the past is a continual challenge in close relationships. This was especially the case with a friend's first spouse. Knowing that she was very ill, my friend began thinking and praying for her and her daughters. Her son-in-law called one morning at 3:30 AM to announce her passing. Quieting the mind he opened his soul to her requesting a visit with her to resolve the old problems.

Within a short time the deceased spouse in spirit appeared as real as life itself. Young and beautiful she stood at the base of the bed. She was full of love and joy. Without speaking words they communicated mind to mind. Their entire life together was reviewed very quickly. They came to realize that all of their experiences were for the good even though very difficult to understand at the time. They forgave each other for all that had been said and done in distress. They both felt peace within their souls and realized they were meant to be together for the time they shared. There was even an awareness they had known each other in a previous lifetime. They freely expressed their gratitude and love for each other and found peace with each other.

It is never too late to ask for help to heal, to forgive and to love another, no matter how much time has passed.

Relationships With Ourselves

The relationships within ourselves include how we relate to our body, emotions, mind and spirit. Learning how to take care of our body is essential to being able to rely on it. Unfortunately we usually do not appreciate its needs until it becomes sick or injured. In the loss of function we learn the role it plays in our health and well-being. Checking in with the body helps us maintain a healthy relationship with it. Asking its preferences in choosing healthy food and exercise elicits cooperation from it. There are thousands of chemical events occurring every day that we do not notice but are necessary for the vitality and support the body needs for its health and healing. Appreciating these many quite automatic functions is an excellent way to start the day. "I love and appreciate all you do for me" is easy to say and do. With meaning, it has an impact like anyone hearing a word of praise.

Relating to our body of feeling plays a great role in learning to relate to others. Our expressions of kindness, compassion, courage and cheerfulness are keys to nurturing a relationship with our own hearts that always precedes relating to the hearts of others. Eventually we learn the value of recognizing small acts of helpfulness and support to ourselves and others. These feelings connect us to the source from which they come. The ability to recognize the good we do and the honest efforts to do the right thing also arises from within. We are meant to be our own best cheerleader and are capable of it.

Findhorn is an exceptional farm in Northern England. It was founded over 30 years ago for the purpose of demonstrating the abundance of nature's resources when properly honored and served. The growth in produce has been extraordinary in size, quality and reproducibility. Most of all the spiritual messages received by the founders provide guidelines for how to work with others in meaningful ways. One of the comments that especially struck me when I first heard one of its founders speak was what the participants are encouraged to say when thanked for work well done: "I'm so glad you noticed!" Although it initially struck me as arrogant it has become a statement of truth that I pass on to others, especially for those who need to notice the effort they make. We often deserve better recognition than we receive but must acknowledge it and accept it when given.

The source of good within deserves to be honored and thanked often. Blaming others for lack of recognition is a sign of missing the source from which our good efforts come. Learning how to support ourselves also prevents unnecessary discord with family, friends, co-members of groups to which we belong and authorities of various kinds. Albert Schweitzer said it well: "It is best not to expect anything from others. Only from ourselves should we expect what we need. That way whatever we receive from others is a gift."

Our relationship with the mind is also worth pursuing. It is the source of many tools and skills including the abilities to organize our life, plan for the day and prepare for the future. It is with the mind that we analyze pros and cons to make a decision and choose the best course to take in a relationship. It is the mind that accesses higher perspectives. As we work with it we become more aware of creative sparks of imagination and innovation. Each day can be more than yesterday if we disconnect from the autopilot and pay attention to the mindful pilot. As we make the effort to awaken the higher mind we can be led to a greater sense of exploring the possible and discovering the unimaginable goodness that we are.

Beyond the mind is the source of its own vitality, the indwelling life and the will to live. Its name is less important than its function which is to fill our life with meaning and purpose and the energy to pursue them. The inner life has an agenda of lessons to learn so that we eventually master the good that can be done through us. We are each unique and have something special to add to the lives of those around us. The closer the relationship we have to the source within the more likely we will find what we have to offer and the will to express it consistently. The spirit within is our potential best friend and our best companion. It is kind and loving though much more interested in what we learn and give than the comforts in which we indulge.

The relationships within ourselves lead us to a healthy body, heart, mind and spirit. As these are developed to work well together we become an integrated person, connected to our inner missions and consistently able to fulfill them. With such an alignment we are able to mobilize healing and wholeness.

Chapter 12

How to Expose and Expel Resistance to Healing

Healing energy is available to us at all times. Being alive and awake means having the potential for calling forth healing energy. Our state of mood and mind determines our effectiveness in invoking the help we may need. However our mood and mind can also get in the way. We can just as easily obstruct the healing flow by dwelling on negative or destructive ways of feeling and thinking. It is necessary to recognize the ways we obstruct healing to motivate ourselves to stop doing so and choose to do what is better.

The most common cause of not healing is not following suggestions for treatment given. This is an ancient problem in medicine and is called the compliance issue. Approximately 50% of people do not take medication the way it is prescribed, which may not be so bad at times. There is now a growing list of ways to motivate people to do better. One of the simplest is reminder calls by office staff which is time consuming but effective. The message to each of us should be that if we structure reminders to ourselves we can develop more consistent ways to implement treatment suggestions given.

I am quite aware of the fact that some people don't comply because they disagree or have an adverse reaction to medication or financial restraints limiting medication usage and treatment procedures. The real problem is when these are not issues. It affects the best of us even when given an effective plan in which we believe.

Comply and Heal

At the pain clinic I had a minister patient with an acute back pain injury. He came to me after seeing an orthopedic surgeon who recommended surgery. He was asking for a second opinion. I reviewed the situation, performed a brief exam and discussed my view that surgery had less than a 50% chance of working. It was clear to me this was not an emergency and there were several things he could do to enhance healing long before surgery should be considered. He was glad to hear my suggestions for healing.

He began a better anti-inflammatory diet and supplements. He returned for a few acupuncture treatments that provided some relief. A few weeks later he declared that he was definitely much better and quite enthused about his recovery. I asked him what made the difference. He proudly proclaimed that just the week before he started the swimming program that we had agreed on the first visit several weeks before. He continued to recover well and did not need surgery. Compliance finally kicked in and made the difference. Accepting a treatment program and following it often leads to healing. As long as we are moving in a healing direction we are improving.

Anger Will Make You Worse

The most common moods that obstruct healing are fear, doubt, worry and anger. They steal our attention and attract energy of a similar nature. When I first see a patient with chronic pain it is necessary to review the history and the sequence of events that led to the current problem. Often in the telling the story people have more pain. Re-living the onset and subsequent frustration reawakens the fear of not healing, of a future with pain and disability, and it worsens the pain. When that happens it is also clear evidence how we worsen our conditions by the mood we choose or too easily re-indulge.

One day I was running a few minutes late. I invited the next patient in to the main room I use. As I was about to start the appointment the previous patient re-entered the office with her dog. She wanted me to meet her dog who meant a great deal to her. Actually she had raised German Shepherds a few years before but was unable to keep up with the demands of continuing to do so. She knew that we had a Shepherd as well. So, for just a few more minutes I greeted her canine companion. She was a very friendly and well-trained and I thanked her for the chance to do so.

The next patient had a chronic low back pain problem. Within a few minutes I reached the point where I began to ask questions about a pain profile. This consists of five measures that give an excellent though subjective assessment of the severity of pain on the whole function of the body and the mood. I asked how much the pain condition was affecting the mood state and specifically how much depression was present most of the time because of it. One hundred is the point of not wanting to live any further, 50% was half of that and 10% only a small amount.

The patient then asked, "How about anger? Why don't you ask about anger?" To which I said "OK, how much anger do you have?" She said "Well, I have a lot more after waiting for the doctor to pet a dog instead of seeing me." By the time we started I was about 20 minutes behind the scheduled time of her appointment.

It became quite apparent this person had a serious problem with herself. She was very depressed and angry. I remembered an old friend and mentor who warned me about certain kinds of people and how he learned to confront them. His saying was "Sorry, I can't help you. I don't want to be in your scrap book of failures." I didn't say that but did tell her that I didn't think I was the right doctor for her. She was concerned I would charge her for the visit anyway since we did have her credit card and do charge for those who do not give us a 24 hour notice before canceling. I reassured her that would not be the case and ended the appointment. Soon after she left she returned and said, "I don't want to see you either." I suspect that her back pain will not improve much until she heals the causes of her anger.

I heard of one orthopedic surgeon who always asked his patients with back pain, "Why are you angry? Who are you angry with?" I recently asked a patient with chronic headaches these same questions. Her response was a surprised look followed by "How did you know? My husband said something very annoying to me just before the headache began."

Anger isolates us from the common sense we need to figure out how to take care of ourselves. We often know what to do, how to handle stress and how to relate to the people with whom we interact. But when we overreact with anger and then fuel it with a feeling of unfairness and insult we make it worse. In doing so we limit the insight we need to figure out how we contributed to the mess in the first place and how to reverse it. Expressing the anger by itself is more likely to make things worse than better. In a controlled setting guided by a trained counselor anger can be healed. The antidotes to anger include patience, a thoughtful review and readiness to forgive self and others. For some the healing choice is to find courage to confront the real cause within self.

Stop Being Stupid

It is not just what we need to start doing to be healthy and well; it is also a matter of what we need to stop doing. People who are overweight need to eat the right foods and stop eating the wrong foods. Those with back pain need to learn healthy exercises to strengthen the back and stop doing activities that worsen it. Many of us need to learn a variety of healthy feelings and moods and unlearn harmful ones.

Overreacting to fears, doubts and worries erodes our self confidence and new plans to establish healthy habits of feeling and thinking. As we seek more peace of mind and heart we need to be willing to stop annoying ourselves with blaming and complaining about all the things wrong about this person, that group or our own body. As we seek better relationships with those around us we need to give up remembering all the petty differences and disagreements we had with them. What we give up is sometimes more important than what we add.

A woman came to see me with chronic fatigue. She was peri-menopausal but had normal blood tests for many hormones. Nonetheless, her adrenal tests were low normal, a common occurrence and reason enough to recommend supplements to optimize function and vitality. I wrote several suggestions including details how to use a liquid adrenal product. Several weeks later I received an angry letter saying that she followed instructions closely, especially with the liquid adrenal for two weeks without seeing any results. She then went to an endocrinologist who put her on hormone replacement and is now feeling wonderful.

When I reviewed the suggestions written out for her I saw that the last suggestion given was to return in two weeks, that if the adrenal gland supplement and the other suggestions don't help we would discuss the use of hormone replacement. She followed some of the suggestions but missed the follow-up to return in two weeks to re-assess the situation. It may have saved her several weeks of waiting and suffering to do so and a consultation with a gynecologist. The original plan with a designed evaluation may have worked. When all else fails re-consider the advice given. If the device doesn't work be sure it is plugged in.

A middle-aged woman came in for a review of her medical status. As she sat in the chair it broke apart. I was dismayed, gathered up the pieces and brought in a new chair. We finished our discussion including an order for blood tests and arrangements for a complete examination. Two weeks later I received a letter saying that she was very upset over my reaction to the broken chair, that I did not show any sympathy for her incident and that I was lucky that she was not in the suing mind because many others would have done so for the potential harm that could have occurred. She also said that she did not plan to see me again.

I reviewed the notes of her visit and my memory of it. She was overweight but not seriously so. However she did sit down rather heavily, and I'm sure that led to the breaking of the chair. I have had several people sit in that chair over the last twenty years many much heavier than she and the chair had never so much as creaked. In reconsidering her visit it became apparent that she did not want to be responsible for the damage she had done, that she chose to blame me for an unfortunate event. Her load of anger and resentment took over with this relatively very minor event. Instead of picking herself up and figuring out what happened she chose to complain. Blaming will often add to the problem, obstruct healing and limit the options available.

How often do we allow our reaction to an event worsen our circumstances far more than the event itself? If it happens more than occasionally that is too often. The challenge is to use such a pattern of events as reason to review the need to cleanse ourselves of the continuing concerns we carry within. The emotional baggage of unresolved anger, frustration, disappointment and hatred is harmful. The straw that broke the camel's back is an old saying about a universal truth still unfolding. The solution is to reassess every day who we are, what we stand for and how to heal the past. We need to reconnect often with our ideal self, our source of loving kindness and forgiveness. We need to awaken it, bath in it and feed it to the rest of who we are. The energy of goodwill and gratitude can help us prevent bad habits from forming.

Not Guilty

The habit of overly criticizing self and others is a deep one and affects far too many of us. A few years ago a new thought church picked up an idea from one of its ministers. It expanded on the wearing of a bracelet to promote a cause, usually in sympathy for a serious illness such as AIDS and other types of cancer. This minister began to suggest that we wear a band to remind ourselves not to complain and be critical. He suggested a commitment of 1-3 months. The movement spread quickly in his church and then many others. It was encouraged at the church I attend. The minister and many others found it very helpful and re-dedicated themselves more than once to an extended period of "fasting from blaming." Simple reminders do make a difference.

Henry Rucker was a minister who consulted patients at the Pain and Health Rehabilitation Center when I worked there. He had a wonderful ability to engage patients quickly with his charm and reassuring ways. One of his favorite talks was on guilt. He would elaborate on how we hold our mistakes in front of us and never let them go like badges of sin and shame that are unforgivable. He would then pass out buttons for each person in the room on which was written in bold letters, "Not Guilty." He would talk about how to remove the guilt, move out of the past into the present, accept the reality of who we are, and make it better.

Guilt is overdone by many. We have a tendency to obsess and never let go of a bad decision, lapse of civility, crudeness or rudeness. We certainly should review our mistakes on a regular basis. We often need to learn how to do better, be kinder, more considerate and more sensitive to those around us. There are many ways to overcome mistakes of behavior and decisions that cause painful consequences that may continue for many years. Some guilt is necessary to honor our conscience that knows right from wrong. Condemnation that extracts a pound of flesh on a daily basis is harmful and must be stopped to re-establish a healthy flow of healing energy. The more sensitive and conscientious we are the more vulnerable we may be to self-rejection. The antidote to guilt is sincere remorse for the harm done and a new dedication to heal and learn from it.

Blaming and Complaining

I was surprised to hear that Dr. Bernie Siegel is accused of making people feel guilty. Dr. Siegel was a Yale surgeon for many years. Due to his compassion for those with cancer he became dedicated and very effective at teaching ways to help them overcome the fear and depression that often accompanies the diagnosis and prognosis of serious cancer. He has written books, given many seminars and appeared on many talk shows including Oprah Winfrey. His main contribution to cancer treatment is developing an intensive treatment program that encourages insight and inspiration. He states that at least 15% of people with serious metastatic cancer have a chance to overcome it with self-reflection and self-renewal efforts. That is a huge contribution compared to conventional medicine.

Many professionals in the medical and psychology field do not agree that we bring on disease, especially cancer. Many believe that it is an accident. But is this how life works? There are accidents at times. We get caught up in the imperfections of life and people's neglect of themselves and those around them. However much disease and especially chronic serious disease such as cancer can often be found to have contributing roots within ourselves. The wonderful benefit of realizing this is that we can also mobilize ways to heal ourselves. This insight recaptures a sense of control and self-awareness that does lead to healing, at times dramatically.

Dr. Siegel is not making people feel guilty because they have cancer. Those who accuse him of doing so have not grasped the concept of how disease works. They are not willing to accept the fact of how disease can be triggered by inner problems that go unresolved. Dr. Siegel teaches people how to love themselves. In the process of learning about love people learn where they did not do so. They feel the pain of fear, self-rejection and rejection of others and the consequences of such choices. Most of all, learning how to love ourselves and those around us liberates the energy of love. Love heals the mind, heart and the body, no matter how sick it may be. Love expels resistance to healing. Blaming and complaining is often an excuse to avoid facing ourself, accepting who we are and the work that can be done to add healing love.

"I Am Sorry" Works

Apologizing triggers the energy of forgiveness. Sincere remorse cannot always be extended to the person or people we have offended. We can express sorrow and regret within ourselves in our hearts to those we slighted or harmed. We can forgive ourselves for our behavior and renew our attention to carefulness, greater respect and greater support of others. We can extend ourselves to be more helpful and reassuring to those around us and thereby undo some of the old acts of awkwardness or flagrant insult.

"I am sorry" is a healing phrase especially when infused with a genuine awareness of the need to do better. However, it often just begins the process. Additional steps are also needed. We need to accept the forgiveness available and then take it deep within ourselves to all the incidents related to the problem. Forgiveness is completed when accompanied by a new willingness to re-engage with others with greater kindness, understanding and dedication.

One of the most difficult experiences I caused was when I mistakenly injected a child with his mother's medication. The child was receiving an unusual innovative intravenous treatment from Germany that required a piggy back infusion. The mother was also suffering from a severe migraine and asked to receive a medication injection. Unknowingly I gave the child her dose of medication that quickly caused a sedating effect. I quickly realized the mistake and called the emergency department of the hospital. The physician on call said to call paramedics, wait for them and not to drive the child directly to the hospital so that treatment could be initiated more rapidly. The mother panicked, took her son in the car and sped off to the emergency room. I dismissed my final two patients and headed off to the emergency room just in case I could be of help to verify what happened.

While driving I was quite aware that the mother might not want to see me and insist I leave the premises. I prayed for help for the child to be saved from major distress and to help me drive safely to the hospital. When I arrived I was readily allowed in and found the room of the child and mother. The mother quickly hugged me, grateful for joining them and we sat together for an extended period of time. An intensivist pediatrician attended the child and we waited to see how he would do. Fortunately, he recovered very well suffering only a brief drowsiness that passed without complication.

I was very grateful the mother was so willing to forgive me. This would not have been easy for many. She provided me with a striking experience of the power of acceptance and forgiveness. I also was very grateful for the invisible forces that may have helped us out as well. Sincere remorse and forgiveness expel errors of judgment and resistance to healing.

What To Add To Healing

What counts toward healing is what we add more than what we expel. Some people attack the cause of disease assuming once that is gone health will move in and take over. Once the pain is gone health is re-established. Once the excess weight is gone good health will be present. Once the depression is gone happiness will reign. Of course this oversimplifies the problem. We are much more than an illness or disease. We are a body of emotion, mind and spirit.

Eliminating what is not working does not guarantee that healthy feelings, ideas or hopes are then present. These must be built individually on their own one at a time. Physically we need to add good habits of diet, exercise and relaxation. Fresh fruits and vegetables, fish and fowl and a variety of healthy foods is the goal. Exercise must be regular and sufficiently challenging to stimulate the heart and blood vessel system to optimize nutrient distribution and metabolic waste elimination.

Emotionally we need to add calmness, confidence, kindness and cheerfulness. These expressions help us maintain a sense of poise and patience while we interact with the people and situations that occur. Enriching our relationships with caring consideration feeds them so that we build friendships that increase our enjoyments and delights. The more social connections we have the more support there is for the difficulties that arise. The kinder we are the more that others willingly share goodwill towards us. The more courage we express the more likely we will confront our challenges instead of retreat from them and the more we will embrace opportunity instead of miss it.

Mentally we need to add goals and projects that honor our major missions in life. We identify our missions by accepting the primary obligations we have chosen. Certainly self-care and self-support are primary. At times close family and friends are the first priorities. Many of us are led to gaps we can fill, needs of our community that call us to respond and leadership positions that we can take on. With help from our higher self we can often find important work to do and loving service to provide. In these ways we add to the life around us, drawing forth the good available to us and making it more available to those in need. Healing energies flow to those engaged in meaningful activities.

Spiritually there is always room to grow and expand. We grow by learning about our source of health and it is continually expressing reassurance, resilience and joy. We grow by expanding our concept of those around us adding an awareness of the strengths of their inner being. Our soul is committed to a broader world view to add perspective and patience as part of our contribution to it. As we commune with its presence we see life through its eyes, how to expel resistance to healing and mobilize the power to heal.

Chapter 13

The Healing Energy of Work Well Done

Work is the wellspring of our lives. It is the means whereby we engage in the business of life, the raising of family, and many kinds of relationships. Work is the way we support ourselves and our family enabling us to provide the basic ingredients of food, clothes, childcare and transportation. It used to be both simpler and harder. We were hunters and gatherers spending most of the time hunting, digging, farming, cleaning, preparing and storing the fruits of our hard labors. In these times a much smaller number of us are actually involved in growing, planting, processing, and delivering basic food nutrients. Now there has become multiple ways to earn a living. The complexity of society has freed up time for many of us to learn many other skills of living that help enrich society and contribute to our community in helpful ways.

As a family physician I have provided services to many who can no longer work. Disability is rarely consciously planned or desired. Accidents and illnesses occur due to a variety of reasons including an imperfect society, carelessness, lack of training and stressful distraction. Diseases happen and they interfere with work and, at times, end it. In particular chronic illness erodes self-confidence, a sense of accomplishment and responsibility. It often leads to further disease, depression and the loss of the ability to develop and maintain relationships.

There is a great deal of literature that documents how individuals malinger after injury and do not want to return to work. My experience is that this is rare, not common, though it does happen. After a weekend of not working, Monday always takes some time to readjust to a full pace of work. After a vacation of only a week, the routine of working takes even longer to re-engage. What are the struggles after several weeks or months of not working or having to return to work with incomplete recovery? Pain, weakness and lack of confidence commonly erode the capacity to be effective at work and at home. Full health is necessary for full work ability.

Work is healing because it provides an opportunity to be constructive and useful in a variety of ways to ourselves and others. Many feel that their job is not this way, that work is drudgery, boring and unfulfilling. Most do not enjoy their job or those with whom they work. Too many resent for whom they work and the conditions under which they work.

However, there are more opportunities available than we are usually aware. Interacting with others forces us to refine and expand our skills to deal with a wider range of problems. Engaging in diverse relationships allows us to learn what other people face. We are not alone and life is rich with unfolding ways to grow.

Work activates all of who we are in body, emotions and mind. Physically it stimulates our senses to be more alert and our body to act in productive ways. Emotionally work requires us to interact with others exposing us to a wide range of states from worry, timidity and stubbornness to kindness, caring and courage. The variety of feelings experienced leads us to opportunities to evaluate our own emotional landscape and assess what works from what does not. Mentally we are stimulated by facing challenging problems that force us to be creative with what is possible. Work propels us to prioritize our concerns, use time efficiently and confront problems directly.

Work engages us in helping others. Interacting with others inspires us to be caring and compassionate which connects us to the spirit of healing energy. The opportunity to help others often goes beyond the skills of our job. One patient reported the following story.

"Recently my wife was diagnosed as having a tumor in one of her sinus cavities, the size of a ping pong ball it turned out. It was pushing precariously close to her optic nerve and carotid artery. A local ear, nose and throat specialist had surgically removed tissue for a biopsy that turned out to be benign, or so it was thought at the time. We were referred to a well-known surgeon at the USC University Hospital for further examination and likely surgery.

"During the visit In Los Angeles, the surgeon raised serious question as to whether the tumor was in fact benign. She thought it likely was not. That was the first red flag. Furthermore, she recommended that the tumor be surgically removed the following week, cancelling a previously scheduled surgery to accommodate my wife. That was another red flag. It was then, when the doctor stepped away for a minute, my wife burst into tears. Both of us were both clearly feeling a greater sense of urgency.

"In the meantime, the surgeon ordered a second CAT scan and MRI for that very day, to get a closer look at what we were dealing with, along with a chest X-ray and other pre-op blood work and interviewing that were pre-requisites for surgery. That is when the scramble began. Just finding your way around a hospital can be daunting. All I really wanted to do at that point was get out of there and drive home as soon as possible. I kept thinking of the freeway traffic getting heavier and heavier, the longer we waited. I felt trapped. But we were no longer on Pacific Time; we were on hospital time.

"I can't remember where I was going by myself in the hospital elevator, but I do recall a nurse carrying a tray of medical paraphernalia. As the elevator door opened she asked me how my day was going, 'Hectic,' I replied. I could hear the shakiness in my voice. I briefly explained the situation.

"Now, I know this nurse was in a hurry to get somewhere. Nurses are always in a hurry to get things done. But this one stopped to help me catch my breath and reassure me that my wife and I were at the right place, receiving the expert care that was needed. She didn't rush off. Instead she paused and was present with me just long enough to help me calm down a little and for a moment, at least, experience my own personal healing.

"I have remembered that nurse many times since, thinking to myself that she did not have to speak to me. She did not have to stop for a moment or two to talk. She could have just kept on going. Thinking of her still has a calming effect on me. Months have passed. My wife's tumor is gone. So are the feelings of anxiety and the sense of urgency. The tumor turned out to be a rare one, but luckily benign. We still visit the USC Hospital for follow-up. And, we are still in those good hands mentioned by the nurse on the elevator, including her own!"

Saying the right thing at the right time is the real goal of loving service. Being skilled, dedicated and attentive to the moment are the hallmarks of work well done. A word of concern, kindness and optimism may go much further than we see or realize.

Finding A Higher Purpose

The higher purpose of work is to serve the larger group to which we belong. There are various degrees at which this occurs. There is the story of a fellow traveling through a region. He came upon a large group of people involved in a major construction project. He asked the first person what he was doing, to which he replied, "I am earning a living, now move on, I am busy here and must get this done." As the traveler moves further he asked another what he was doing. The man responded, "I am supporting my family, my wife and children; this is good job that I like doing. Now don't interfere with the work I must do." The traveler proceeded further asking a third worker in the same field, "What are you doing?" To which the worker paused, looked up and said. "Me? Why, I am building a cathedral."

Of course they were all doing the same kind of work. What was different was the purpose chosen of the work being done. In many circumstances most of us are primarily serving self. Some are serving a family and extended family. And some are serving a grand vision of a larger whole. Although the groups of activity in which we are now involved are usually complex we still have choices to grudgingly do our job, consider it as just a way to make a living or identify with a larger mission. The more we can grasp the higher nature of the work we do, the more we will be supported in our efforts. The higher vision energizes all those who see it and serve it. The larger perspective is healing physically and psychologically. It connects us to a larger field of support, strength and persistence.

There are work sites that are negative fields of energy. Some groups foster goals that are critical rather than creative, divisive instead of inclusive or aggressive instead of attentive. All can be used to make life better. However, some supervisors and individuals are so self-serving they increase the risk of disease instead of providing sources of support or fulfillment. I have heard many stories from several of my patients of co-worker and management abuse. Legal guidelines help moderate some of the abuse but by the time it can be activated a great deal of suffering has occurred.

There are those who suffer and those who cause suffering in the work place. It is hard to value the work you do in such a situation. However it is worth realizing that the cause of abuse is just as often not the abuser as the one who takes it without action. Speaking up in some manner is necessary. It can be done directly to the individual or creatively around the individual. Occasionally the best thing is to find another job. Most of the time the goal should be to find ways to confront the situation. Learning how to speak up is a necessary skill of living that we all must learn.

The first reason to learn to take a stand is self-preservation and self-respect. Advanced reasons for learning how to confront difficult people is for our own benefit and the health of the company for which we work. A healthy working atmosphere requires decent working relationships among the team whether the office is small or large. The more the many subunits work well together the healthier is the whole. Just as the health of the body requires healthy cells for a healthy organ, and healthy organs for a healthy body, a healthy company requires well functioning individuals and groups of them for the company to be well.

The real challenge in a difficult work situation may be to find ways to persist, to persevere and to thrive. Dedication to a high purpose is often what is missing in work environments and not easily instilled. Such a setting can still be an experience of learning and growing if nothing more than a negative example of what not to do. At times the solution is to stand up and leave. The highest paying job is not necessarily the best one. At other times it is best to accept the circumstances and cultivate the virtues needed. Such a challenge increases the strength to cope in difficult surroundings.

Healing A Dysfunctional Workplace

Strategies for dealing with dysfunctional work settings include the need to work, the truth about what isn't working and ways to build healthy expectations.

The first task is to consider the need to have the job. When there is little opportunity for moving to another job easily it is clear that limiting frustration is essential. Most of us need to learn how to minimize our emotional reactions, and this is an opportunity to do so.

The second step is find the truth about difficulties that arise. Often it seems misinterpretation exaggerates the problem from a minor annoyance into an almost impossible dilemma. Carefully considering the facts and asking for objective verification can help immensely to heal an unfortunate event, or at least re-establish lines of communication and workable relationships.

The third step in healing a difficult work environment is to look for ways to build healthy expectations. Before the workday begins many find it worthwhile to rehearse the day the way they would like it to go. This can include a desire to perform the expected duties well, conscientiously and competently. Most of the day is predictable concerning the most likely stressors and meaningful interactions. Rehearsing a probable encounter in a positive way with a difficult co-worker increases the chance for it to occur that way. Choosing a sense of cooperation contributes to a better possible work relationship even with difficult people. It is more likely to attract the capacity to do so instead of the energy of dismay, distress and disgust.

Sometimes the best way to heal or prevent disease is to leave. Some situations are impossible and the best option is to look for another job. I am amazed at how often people are in such a situation and still drag their feet in creating new opportunities. However, a decision should not be made abruptly unless serious verbal and emotional abuse is present and frequent.

I recall my wife working for a difficult manager who seemed quite unfair and was getting worse. It was a very good position for her at the time. She considered leaving to get out of the very uncomfortable relationship. I advised waiting and watching awhile longer to see if the situation evolved to her benefit. She agreed to do so and within only a few weeks the head of the department committed a serious misjudgment resulting in her quick departure. At times that is the healing needed. I have heard this happen more than once. Persistence can pay off in the worst of situations.

I had a patient who worked at a large institution of learning. She was transferred at one point to work for an executive who had a bad reputation in her staff relations. She followed her boss's instructions, worked diligently and was always on time. She seemed to be considered competent until criticisms began to increase. At a certain point it was apparent that her boss was being very unfair in assessing her performance, distorting requests made and obsessing about minor mistakes. She appealed to the personnel department who sided with her boss. As she became physically ill I suggested she begin counseling. When she did not improve I suggested she begin to look for a different job. She resisted for several months but eventually was forced out. Once she was free of the influence of the abusive boss she improved rapidly. There is a time to fight and a time to move on.

Confronting authority can bring healing to a whole organization. A patient came to me with a shoulder pain. We tried various treatments that only had moderate benefits. At a certain point I asked about the stress in her life. She was a teacher and said that her main stress was the principal at the school. As I found out more it became clear that the principal was playing favorites, changing rules without notice and generally treating most of the teachers unfairly. I told her that the shoulder pain was her responsibility regardless of the behavior of the principal. She was upset with this comment and I wasn't sure she would return.

She did return. At the request of her lawyer she asked for a letter of support. My letter served its purpose. She eventually was able to convince the board of trustees about the multiple abuses inflicted on the faculty. The board decided to fire the principal and assistant principal, re-establishing good working conditions for the staff. Confronting authority is not easy and the mission to do so should be planned carefully.

Loving The Work You Do

"Work is love made manifest" Kahlil Gibran said. The more we love the work we do the more likely we will receive the support we need to do it well. The main support available to us all is the depth and beauty of our own heart, mind and spirit. Loving the work we do begins with appreciating the work we have. We have to learn how to enjoy the people with whom we work. We need to emphasize what we like about it more than what we do not. Ideally we identify with the larger missions of the work we do, who it serves and why.

Raising a family is a continuous job from morning to night. It requires all the skills of living to do it well. It requires more than saying we love our kids and family. It requires sacrificing self care, sleep, good diet and exercise as part of the work that must be done. Patiently attending to the impulses of children pushes us to the maximum of our abilities and forces us to reach within ourselves for determination to persist. There are celebrations, precious moments and joys that make it all worthwhile. However it is work. It is made easier when going well but more often the high moments must be pondered often to handle the difficult times. Loving our children is easy when they are sleeping and well but harder when awake and ill. This is when they need more attention than we want to give. The challenge is to learn how to love them under all circumstances. In the process we learn the deeper sides of the many faces of love, devotion, tolerance for differences, forgiveness, patience and long-term commitment.

It helps immensely to learn how to enjoy the people with whom we work. For many this is a mutual goal. For others we need to toughen our ability to tolerate annoyances. Fostering awareness of shared goals and generating cooperation is a sign of success.

One of my mentors has been Edgar Cayce the pioneer of American holistic medicine. A phrase he said often in advising people how to lead their life was to *"seek to be a channel of blessings to others."* To be a blessing means to be helpful, to make a difference and to be part of something larger than self. When we love being a parent we raise our children for the future and instill them with the strengths they will need.

Loving the work we do means that we see value in it. The main value of the work we do is in increasing the interest, enthusiasm and optimism it brings to our own life and that of others, however small that may be. The groundskeeper for a friend of mine has more than once made a huge impact on her. When a recurring plumbing problem interrupted a long weekend he was available and able to fix it quickly. She trusted him and his assessment and came to trust his opinion about things other than his maintenance skills might warrant. Any job that is mastered well can be a healing experience for those we serve and ourselves.

Loving the work we do needs to be awakened every day. We do this by loving our capacity to perform it and consistently looking for ways to improve it. It helps to imagine the work unfolding as expected, with creative moments of loving what we do, those we serve and the space we fill.

Loving the work we do mobilizes the power to heal ourselves and those with whom we work and live.

Awaken the Genius Within

Chapter 14

Restoring the Magic of Memory

Memory is the function of the mind in how we process and store events, interactions and the energy of them. The common definition of memory is the ability to remember names, dates, and details of events, conversations and activities. Although these are useful functions memory is much more. It is a complex capacity for organizing not only what happens to us but also our reactions and the array of energies associated with them. Our reactions reach into many areas of feeling, thought and willfulness from the recent and distant past.

In some respects our memory capacities are like the workings of a post office. It receives mail from a wide range of people and organizations, sorts it out according to destination and then connects it to the appropriate distribution centers. Of course the post office is much more than the physical letters, packages, boxes, buildings and vehicles. It is also the people at various levels of skill, supervision and authority from simple to complex. So, too, our memory banks are multidimensional. We function at physical, emotional, mental and spiritual levels with energy messages moving back and forth from one dimension to another.

Our sensory system receives impulses from the five wonderful senses. It sends the messages along an intricate array of nerve branches toward the central processing sites of the brain where decisions are considered for further action. Physical events register within the cells and organs of the body. They remember a wide range of sensations that become part of the reflex reaction instinct. A single odor of a favorite flower or perfume, taste of a delicious food or drink, the sound of a familiar piece of music or sight of a friend, sets in motion multiple connections of memories. Although initial sensations register in appropriate storage banks in the brain, individual cells retain memories as well. Sensations trigger feelings of various kinds as well as thoughts of previous similar experiences.

Our emotional bodies have their own patterns of reactions and memories depending on the experiences we have accumulated. There are grooves of fears, doubts, worries, enjoyments, hopes and desires. These accumulated patterns become paths that we slip into easily which is beneficial for simple tasks but not for others. Just as most of us do not want to play the same music over and over, so too we should not want to keep replaying old habits that are detrimental. Instead we need to be looking for new experiences, associations and meanings in current events of our life. A dynamic active memory grows more by exploring new expressions than by reviewing old ones over and over.

Healthy memories are helpful but unhealthy ones may not be. Unresolved experiences are especially harmful to the memory like a scratch on an old record. It plays the scratch that is noise, not music. Replaying memories of fear, frustration and distress obscure the healthier parts of who we are. Choice is always available although the deeper the groove the more difficult it may be to create a new focus of attention. Eventually they must be worked through, smoothed out and harmonized with the rest of who we are. All the notes of our life are meant to be part of a grand symphony. This is the goal and the possibility toward which we strive. It does not happen by continually replaying only the discordant notes, the scratches and scrapes of life.

Our memory is a marvelous complex dynamic process of continual action. The more we are aware of its function the more we can tap into its rich store of experience for new creative expressions and decisions. Our memory is meant to be a major resource for guidance, direction and healing. This resource is especially activated when remembering our missions in life, a major source of power for healing and wholeness.

A Healthy Memory

Remembering many facts, figures, names and dates only touch the surface of our memory banks. Far more important is the quality of memories we call upon and put to use.

We use our memories for healthy functions every day. How we dress, groom, and prepare ourselves for the day's routine is a common function. It serves a purpose in presenting ourselves to others in a decent, civil manner. When we go about our work each day we usually pick up where we remember we left off the day before and hopefully make further progress. When we interact with others we stimulate memories of the last encounter and maybe key ones related to the point of the meeting and discussion.

More complicated tasks unfold in a similar way. An example is how we raise our children. We learn from what we experienced from our parents or those close to us. We can imitate what we learned or add new ways of handling similar problems that occur. Memory is always a complex of images, feelings and actions. We may only recall the way a diaper is changed or the baby is fed but what is also activated is the attitude and presence of mind with which it is done. The more we awaken our own true sense of self the more we will express our higher presence of selfless devotion and dedication. Although we learn from others we build only on the memory of our own experience. The real bricks come from our own choices of feeling, thinking and aspiration.

A healthy memory is one in which we use the past to help us through the day. It is a healthy use of memory when we have a big decision to make and access the best decisions we have previously made. From these we can also review the sense of rightness we have learned, how to identify it and recreate in a new way.

A healthy memory continues to extract meaning from major events and relationships of the recent and distant past. It helps us assess the status of current opportunities and the presence or absence of ingredients necessary to pursue them. It has peak events readily available for inspiration and new direction. A healthy memory remembers turning points, roads not taken and why they may be available now. It remembers how we recovered from mistakes, awkward expressions and missed opportunities.

A healthy memory is often aware of the missions of the soul for growth, learning and ways to help others. This is the temple in which we dwell. And it is continually capable of positive change.

Memory Misuses

Too many of us use memory to review the traumas and tragedies we have experienced. If there is a bad weather day it is an occasion to review the worst weather days we remember. If there is a personal illness the worst we know of it is reviewed and how difficult it has been. If there is a natural catastrophe we review its devastating effects and those of other natural disasters we remember. The value in these memories is how we learned to protect ourselves, adapt to difficulty, survive and thrive in spite of them not just the turmoil of them.

The misuse of memory should be considered a cause of disease. When fears and worries are awakened each day they build an intensity that attracts more of the same. It is like growing a garden and then going out of our way to water the weeds instead of the food and flowers that are there. As we review the feelings of insecurity, frustration and failure we magnify the worst within us. The dominant emphasis of our difficult past may diminish our self-esteem and lead to a poor self-image. Over time we can lose connection to the healthy experiences of patience, tolerance and forgiveness which in turn leads to developing a vortex of depression and despair. These often lead to a breakdown of nerve, hormone and immune changes that increase our risk for a wide range of disease. This is how we create disease. There are consequences to the choices of memories on which we choose to focus.

I recall a patient who attended the Pain Clinic. She relayed the story of an old memory she replayed many, many times. At a certain point in her life she began to observe how she could do things better than others. She developed the nasty habit of muttering the phrase to herself "I could do that standing on one leg." One day, years later, she noticed a lump on her leg. She went to her physician who diagnosed a serious cancer that required amputation of her leg. Eventually she learned that sneering at others created a serious focus for disease. She poured her scorn into a specific site on the body that attracted energy of a similar nature, a very destructive one. She came to this insight and shared it with all of us in a group. She was grateful that she could now understand what she did not know before. To her the cancer was no longer from an unknown cause or just an accident of nature. It came from misdirecting the energies of her heart and mind. Fortunately she also learned the healing effects of a healthy focus. She became quite able to direct the healing energies of forgiveness and growth to herself in positive accepting ways.

The Primary Purpose Of A Healthy Memory

What are your reasons to have a healthy memory? The obvious benefits are to perform the usual functions of the day, of awaking on time, bathing, eating, dressing and behaving appropriately. We review what needs to be done and organize the day so that the main tasks and obligations will be accomplished. Ideally we set aside time at the beginning of the day to recall the higher purposes of our life. If we are raising children it is worth thinking about the best way to help them today. It is worth considering the special needs of each of those entrusted to our care and how we improve them. Some may need a bit more cheer and optimism to overcome sadness. Others may need a little more patience to overcome irritability with friends. Others may benefit with a greater capacity to be assertive instead of timid, or friendly instead of aggressive or enthused instead of grumpy. The memory of how we've expressed these in the past brings them to the front of our memory banks for quick use when ready. What is retrieved is not only the quality of expression but also the energy of it, all of which can be expanded with new intention. The new better intention is the power of healing.

The beginning of the day can be an excellent time to awaken the ideal uses of memory of our major missions. Although one day will not make a great difference in how far we proceed, it can become a day in which we have moved toward our goals instead of simply treading water or sinking further. For some, just getting through the day with less depression is an accomplishment. For others the goal is to advance the top priorities. If there is a challenging event to occur or person to meet asking ourselves certain questions may be helpful. Why are we planning to meet and how can we make it most worthwhile? How can we best prepare for the conversation? What presence of mind and heart do we most want to bring? What do we need to learn from this encounter? What do we have to offer this person or event that is beneficial?

Our higher aspirations and motivations need to be awakened daily for them to flourish. If our day will have turmoil what memories are available to help us be more calm and confident? If our day is likely to be boring and very routine what memories are likely to awaken curiosity and enthusiasm? If our day appears overwhelming how can we call forth the times when we were better organized, more able to prioritize and more likely realize the good person who we are?

Our highest memories are the ways we have made a difference for those around us. Our peak events are usually times when we best recognized the need of another and made our effort to help. This may be a time when we expressed love for the attention of another or felt that love in return. It may be the expression of gratitude given or received. It may be one of the many generous efforts of kindness we saw and felt.

The higher self wants us to remember successes and decisions rightly chosen. We need to be review them often especially when an important decision is approaching. Success is often a result of accumulated effort, persistence and patience. Remembering how we began a certain project and followed through to its completion helps imprint a conscious pattern that we can continue to draw upon when needed. A successful sequence memory can become a powerful reminder of how we are able to handle a complicated situation effectively. It reconnects us to the source of strength and resilience within our own memory banks and the energy with which to do it.

Healing Memories Of Mistakes And Missed Opportunities

We have a conscience for the purpose of being aware of who we are. Our conscience helps us know when we do less than we are able or the opposite of what we expect. There is a capacity within us that knows our obligations and commitments. It is our constant companion, a close ally of our soul. It is a truth seeker within us. Although it is a source of self-criticism it is not a fire and brimstone inner critic that demands perfection unless we make it so.

The inner conscience is designed to help us remember our priorities of the day. It helps us decide what is best from what is not. It can help us organize the day. Its true value depends on the extent to which we exercise it. As we invite its guidance we are made aware of the quality of our expressions, interactions and opportunities to engage our true nature.

The keynote of healing memories is integrity. This is the capacity to be straightforward, genuine and authentic to ourselves. Integrity is the strength of truth that measures the value of our self worth. It helps to ensure that we act on what we hold to be important. Our faith, beliefs and expectations are one thing. The ability to act on them is another. The energy of integrity is a source of healing memories. As we sincerely seek to be true to ourselves we invoke the presence of truth and how to expand it further within us.

The 12-Step program for Alcoholics Anonymous provides an excellent guideline for healing memories. It emphasizes a "fearless inventory of wrongs" which requires us to accept the facts of what we've done poorly or did not do when we could have and should have.

Part of having a healthy conscience is to be fair to ourselves which means to have a balanced view of our shortcomings. Yes, we need to have an honest inventory of our past especially major missteps. Yet we also need to remind ourselves what we've done well, correctly and honestly. If we are overly critical we separate ourselves from the source of healing that will enable us to move on humbler and wiser.

Healing memories of the past begin with identifying an oasis of well-being. We need to have a sense of worth upon which we can draw forth the energy of healing. The web site of well-being contains the memories of what we have done well. However small the good we have done connects us to the source from which they came. This is the energy we mobilized to do the right thing at the right time. The more we review our involvement in the sequence of choices from beginning to end the more we build our confidence and trust in the good within us. This is how we connect ourselves to our own center of well-being.

The center of our well-being is also the source of forgiveness. The spirit of forgiveness is available to all of us. To tap into it we must trust our inner being to respond. To mobilize it requires a sincere appeal for help and a willingness to admit our shortcomings. Keeping it simple, straightforward and to the point invites the energy of forgiveness to enter in and pour forth its healing energy. As we trust the energy of forgiveness to know where to go and follow through with what happens healing occurs.

The Hawaiian prayer of reconciliation says it well: "I love you, I forgive you, please forgive me, thank you." Repeated over and over this appeal can attract the sensitivity and depth of what there is to forgive, a willingness to learn from what has happened and a dedication to do better.

We must have reasonable expectations. Minor problems do not require ash on the forward, beating of the chest, tearing of the heart and elaborate promises of never happening again. A prior conscious intent to deceive or harm does widen the gap between the good intention to heal and the source of honesty. If there is a chasm between us and the source of sincerity it will require more than simply saying you are sorry. A new better behavior must be chosen that is persistently continued over time for full healing of the problem.

In *The Color Purple,* the main character is played by Whoopi Goldberg. Her husband is very abusive, emotionally, physically and sexually. He is also unfaithful more than a few times. As Celie finally frees herself from him she establishes her real sense of self. She eventually returns to where they lived as an empowered individual with her own strengths upon which to draw. The final scenes show her ex-husband living nearby and coming to visit for a weekly Sunday dinner that she kindly continues to make for him. They treat each other respectfully recognizing the struggles they have come through, the shortcomings in each other, the healthy changes they made and reasons to continue their relationship though with distance between them. This is a sign of real healing. This is a demonstration of how to heal the past.

Missed opportunities need attention as well. These may be healed by paying closer attention to the current obligations we have. Major decisions are usually few and far between. Our ability to do well with what we have prepares us for what is to come. I have missed my share of greater things to do and people to know. Nevertheless I have come to appreciate that this point in time has its own opportunities. As these are considered carefully and conscientiously much good can be done. The roads not taken that may have been better are not forever gone. Each day is a chance to awaken a creative spark to make it interesting and very worthwhile.

How To Increase The Skills Of Remembering

In the physical body, the basic needs for a healthy memory are derived from an optimal exercise regimen, sleep efficiency, healthy diet, and specific supplements for healthy nerve function. Memory occurs at each level of our being, body, heart, mind and spirit. Each requires a different set of suggestions for optimal function.

A diet for the nervous system is similar to a general good diet. The basic ingredients need to be optimal proteins, carbohydrates and fats. They each play a role in the structure of the nerve cell and its function.

Some people can function well on lower protein levels than others. The amounts will vary from one person to another. Some amino acid components are more important than others. The first goal is to have a blood level total protein in the upper half of normal. Even then a specific amino acid profile may be helpful in identifying individual building block deficiencies.

The same is true for the many kinds of fatty acids that provide the lattice network of nerve cell outer membrane. An intact lining membrane ensures optimal nerve cell to cell transmission. The **omega 3 fatty acids** rather than the omega 6, 7, and 9 fatty acids are more likely to be deficient and therefore more likely need to be supplemented.

B12 deficiency has been found to be associated with memory loss especially in the elderly. A basic supplement approach should include healthy amounts of the B vitamin family such as a B complex 100 provides. In addition, extra amounts of B12 and folic acid may be necessary depending on the blood test levels.

Choline has more recently become of greater interest in treating memory loss. It is the building block for acetylcholine which is the most prominent neurotransmitter involved with Alzheimer's Syndrome. Most of the medications for treating it inhibit acetylcholinesterase, the enzyme that breaks down acetylcholine. Taking large amounts of choline can compensate to some degree. Choline is a member of B vitamin complex and is mainly found in eggs and fatty meat. It is estimated that only 2% of postmenopausal women obtain enough in the usual diet.

Acetylcholine is the neurotransmitter most likely to become deficient as memory decreases and other cognitive skills become impaired. There are several medications that prevent its loss and one over the counter supplement called **galantamine.** This is an active component of the snowdrop flower that was referred to in *The Odyssey*, written by Homer 2500 years ago. He used it to reawaken his sailors from the spell of the Sirens, the nasty spirits who were lonely and wanted the men to forget who they were and the mission they pursued so they would stay with them on the island. Many studies have been conducted in its use for those with memory loss and Alzheimer's Syndrome with variable reports of improvement. Benefit occurs in many with mild to moderate memory loss.

For the same reason other **neurotransmitters** should also be tested and most likely supplemented. Serotonin, dopamine, noradrenaline and adrenalin all play a role in nerve function. These have been studied in terms of depression, weight loss and sleep dysfunction each of which affects memory. A spot urine test is the best way to measure their levels in the body. As the precursors to these neurotransmitters are increased the levels of the nerve hormones are too, as well as the functions they provide.

Gradually increasing **5-hydroxy tryptophan (5 HTP)** increases serotonin. Supplements of **tyrosine** increase the level of dopamine and its byproducts of noradrenaline and adrenaline. Because serotonin and tyrosine compete for the same enzyme, they should be taken concurrently, ideally in a 10-1 ratio of tyrosine to 5 HTP.

Most of the **major hormones** of the body are necessary for a healthy memory function. The adrenal, thyroid and gender hormones should each be optimized. Blood, saliva and urine tests can be used to assess current levels. My goal is to improve their levels, usually to the upper half of normal.

The **adrenal hormones** to test include DHEA, pregnenolone and cortisol. DHEA is the most prevalent adrenal hormone and the easiest to test and supplement. Studies verify its ability to increase memory function. Its use should be balanced with whole adrenal gland or hydrocortisone, depending on levels found and symptoms reported. Adverse effects are mild, uncommon and reversible. Pregnenolone was studied for enhancing memory over 50 years ago, but it was not found to be consistent though it may be considered helpful in some situations.

Thyroid hormones commonly decrease as we age and play a major role in memory use. Thyroid panels are readily available, although conventional medicine is concerned mainly when thyroid stimulating hormone (TSH) is abnormal. In addition, the usual treatment is T4, not T3, the assumption being that most people convert T4 to T3 easily. This is unfortunate because function can be improved by reaching more specific upper levels of free T3 and free T4. People over the age of 50 respond better to using both T3 and T4. Overuse can occur resulting in excess stimulation of the intestines, heart or nervous system. These are not common and quite reversible when amounts are gradually increased and symptoms are monitored closely.

Gender hormones include **estrogen, progesterone and testosterone.** They each have a major impact on well-being, energy and nerve-brain function. There is much controversy with their use because of fear of cancer. However risk for cancer can be diminished by assessing family history, regular exams, screening tests and adjusting metabolic breakdown products. The more serious the memory loss concern the greater should be the effort to maximize the use of these hormones. Even modest amounts can have beneficial effects in alertness, concentration and memory abilities.

In addition to diet and supplements, **exercise** plays a major role in memory function. Two simple strength tests measure our risk for vascular problems in the brain. Hand grip strength and pace of walking correlate with stroke and dementia risk. General strength diminishes with age in part because we do not use the muscles we have and also due to decreasing circulation. Aerobic cardio exercise is the best kind of exercise to prevent blood vessel plaque formation and ensure excellent delivery of nutrients to the brain and spine. A good goal guideline is walking one hour per day or a half hour of more vigorous jogging, cycling or swimming.

Sleep efficiency declines as we age. Those with more sleep problems have greater evidence of brain chemical breakdown. Nighttime sleep is when nutrients are delivered to each cell of the body and waste products are best removed for later discharge. Each of the major systems of the body regenerates during the sleep state. The more nighttime interruptions the less restoration occurs. The more sleep we have the greater our nervous system is replenished and ready for a full day's activities.

Although the physical approaches to increasing memory have more studies to support their use the psychological aspects have huge potential for improving brain-mind function. The extent to which we remember is largely based on habits of stimulating the mind to be curious, thoughtful and involved in the issues of our life. Our social life may be the best resource there is for activating our brain, heart and mind.

There are many **mental exercises** for strengthening memory access. These have some value and for those interested should be pursued. They include card games, crossword puzzles and a growing array of computer mind games. The more involved and dedicated we participate in any of these the greater the benefit. The level of intensity and consistency are the determining factors more than any one game or tool. However, creative efforts are continuing to expand ways to challenge the brain and mind.

As we age there is a decreased capacity to remember certain items, names and recent activities. Asking questions after each encounter, program or reading period will help register details for better memory retrieval. Interacting with others in conversation definitely increases the memory of key words, phrases and feelings that are experienced.

Assigning an image to an item to be remembered is an old technique that continues to work for anyone using it. The best images are those that have the greatest meaning, interest or humor associated with them. Once when I forgot the name of a neighborhood magnolia tree and its gorgeous bowls of blossoms I associated the letters M and M that stand for magnificent magnolia. It was never forgotten again. When our son attended a camp at our first get-acquainted meeting with the counselor, he had us go around the circle with our name one time. He then went from one to the next telling us our name, checking himself and impressing us with his remembering about 25 names in a short period of time. He simply assigned each name to a major event from his life and had little trouble remembering them the rest of the week long session.

The best exercise for the memory begins with deciding what you most need to remember. We associate details of names, dates and events with a healthy mind not succumbing to age. I suggest that the hierarchy of needs begins with our highest priorities and the questions we ask ourselves concerning them. Is it just the last conversation you had that you seek to remember or the feelings stimulated during the interaction? Is it just the feelings we have during the day that stimulate a variety of reactions or the questions and challenges in which we are involved? Do we want to remember details of what we hear and read or the capacities to solve problems, to consider underlying intentions, to engage in complex issues and be able to consider consequences of important decisions?

More complex questions about what we cherish in life may lead us even further. What do we need to learn about ourselves to make the most of it today? What do we need to learn to help those who are in our sphere of responsibility? What are the questions that life is asking us to learn about and contribute to solving for ourselves and those around us? What are the ideals toward which we strive?

Curiosity is one of the most important skills of the mind that contribute to a growing memory. Our instinctive curiosity causes gaper's block that slows down traffic because drivers feel compelled to see what happened. As a skill of the mind curiosity is a vital doorway through which many other skills are awakened. To be curious means to frequently observe and wonder what is happening on the surface and behind the scenes. To be curious means to want to know why people say what they do, think what they do and change who they are. To be curious means to ask questions of ourselves, those around us and those we hear and read about. The mind is especially stimulated to answer the questions we ask. The art of asking about the life we live increases our connection to the source from which it comes and the direction in which it is going. Curiosity is a grand doorway to accessing what we know and adding to the memory banks we have. A healthy memory can help us mobilize our healing power.

Steps That Increase Memory

1. A healthy diet that emphasizes adequate protein and omega 3 fatty acids.
2. A vigorous exercise routine that emphasizes head-neck-spine stretching and a one-hour walk equivalent per day.
3. Adequate sleep of 6-8 hours per day.
4. Supplements that may include the following:
   a. B complex 100mg/day.
   b. B12 1mg/day.
   c. Folic Acid 0.8mg/day.
   d. Choline 500mg/meal.
   e. Fish oil 1000mg/meal or Omega 3 fatty acids 1000mg/meal.
   f. Tyrosine and 5 HTP in a 10:1 ratio beginning at 500/50mg per meal.
5. Medications that may include optimal amounts of:
   a. Thyroid medication if indicated.
   b. Adrenal supplements if indicated.
   c. Estrogen and progesterone if needed and appropriate.
   d. Testosterone if helpful and appropriate.
   e. Growth hormone precursors or medication if helpful and possible.
   f. Galantamine as a supplement or medication.
6. A concerted effort to heal past memories of trauma, fear, anger and disappointment.
7. Mental exercise suggestions:
   a. Begin every day remembering the highest priorities.
   b. Expect opportunities to learn, enjoy and help others.

c. Request and expect help from the higher self to make the day active, meaningful and enjoyable.
d. Live the day attentive, flexible, firm, kind and curious,
e. Ask questions as often as possible.
f. At the end of the day review the best thoughts, feelings and events with gratitude and graciousness.
g. Take the best of the day with you to bed for the night.

Chapter 15

How to Discover and Develop Intuition

Intuition is a sense of inner knowing. It is a means of accessing information that goes beyond the physical senses. We have five senses of sight, sound, taste, smell and touch. However these are all physical ways of communicating with the world around us. Intuition is from beyond the body. It can be emotional, mental or spiritual, and the higher the better. The information received is in the form of feelings, thoughts or inspirations. The closer to the source of truth the more accurate and helpful are the hints given.

More commonly intuition is referred to as "a gut feeling", an "ah-ha!" or "a flash of insight." We label it in various ways but the label is not as important as receiving the new input needed. We all have various concerns, conditions and challenges on our plate. Most of the time we are doing the best we can to solve the problems we have. Intuition is how we go beyond the usual way to access awareness. It is helpful to consult those who know more than we do. However, intuition is how we develop our own sense of knowing.

Intuition acts like an in-home mentor. It is smarter though not all-knowing, concerned for our well-being but not primarily responsible for decisions made. It is able to provide a broader perspective and point out pitfalls that may not be noticed. It enables access to our basic set of knowledge and experience as well as a higher perspective and possibility.

I recently saw a patient with a sore throat and flu-like symptoms. On examination he had swollen tonsils with exudate, enlarged lymph nodes of the neck and a very fatigued appearance. He was sick. He had already seen two other physicians who probably see many more patients like this than I. Each of them had done a throat Strep test that was negative. I did one, too, because he had an obvious bacterial infection. Maybe they didn't swab it right and missed the bugs; surprisingly mine was negative also. I thought there was clearly an infection and swabbed the throat for lab identification of the bacteria growing. Sure enough two days later it showed a non-Strep bacterial infection, fortunately easily treated with an antibiotic.

The other physicians told him he had a viral infection and left it at that. Without an antibiotic there was a chance he would have become seriously ill if it progressed. Why didn't they go further? To what extent can we use intuition to diagnose our own physical and psychological problems? When is intuition appropriate to use and when not? How do we activate the intuition available?

Activating Healing Impulses

Intuition is often triggered by asking a question. Yes and no questions are easier to sense and interpret. As we make our choices and options clear we can more easily add to them. Practical ways to improve our health may be to ask ourselves about the foods we consider for our next meal. Can I handle one piece of bread or not? Should I have another serving? Should I have dessert and, if so, which one? Many of us struggle to eat well, especially during the holidays or at our favorite restaurant. Our inner being is dedicated to our health and can help us know which food will digest best, most provide the energy we need and still be enjoyable. We may not like the answer we receive but need to be willing to accept the consequences of not acting on our best behalf. Objectivity is a key to the skillful use of intuition.

Intuition is meant to be used for daily concerns. Exercise is essential for basic health and well-being. Some folks seem to get by with doing little exercise but I see them in the office suffering from not doing enough for far too long. Most people definitely feel better with exercise though it requires obvious effort. We can ask ourselves whether to exercise today or not, which form is best and how to develop the habit of doing it regularly.

Intuition can be reassuring and useful by simply encouraging us to ask someone for help. Occasionally I see a patient in the office who has been having a recent cough or ache. There is a growing concern because it is not going away. Just by making the appointment it sometimes feel better. The reason for feeling better may be because action is being taken to check it out further. The nagging fear of something serious can be connected to a family member or friend having a common symptom that turned out to be cancer. A healthy part of ourselves can suggest the need to act because the fear of a serious problem alone.

At times a more serious problem does occur that can be aided with intuition. I recently met a woman who told me a compelling story about how intuition saved her life. When she was 32 she went to her gynecologist because of left breast pain similar to pre-menstrual breast tenderness. The breast exam was normal but the physician recommended mammograms every 6 months for two years. The results were always the same with some calcification but no suspicious changes over that time. He finally decided to act anyway suggesting, "If you were my wife I would send you to a surgeon to consider a biopsy."

She proceeded to the surgeon who had his own radiology expert for doing mammograms and repeated the x-ray. Again the report was without positive findings. The surgeon overrode these findings and recommended surgery that she had two days later. A small but aggressive breast cancer was discovered and later removed with a total mastectomy and axillary lymph node dissection. She underwent eight months of chemotherapy and five years of tamoxifen. Thirteen years later she is cancer free and very grateful for the physicians who followed their inner sense to look further. To her it was intuition that led her and her physicians to the real diagnosis and successful treatment.

Intuition for Decision Making

Some of the most important decisions I have made have been from intuitive impulses. When I was about 15 years old I remember coming upstairs. My parents were talking in the dining room and looked up as I went by. My dad asked, "What do you think you'd like to be when you get older." We did not discuss my future prior to that and so it was not a common topic. I had not thought much about it but quickly responded that, "I think I'll be a doctor." They seemed satisfied and on I went. That comment did not come from a conscious thought process but out of the blue from my higher mind I suspect. My older brother was in medical school at the time and my mother was a registered nurse. Medicine is in the family so it made it easier to consider. The comment had the hallmarks of intuition, sudden, clear and without obvious consideration.

I attended an in-state university and proceeded to the only medical school there. At the time it was one of only three in the country with a two-year program. We all had to transfer to another school for the last two years for direct patient care training. Most schools could easily work us in because clinical rotations through the various specialties are more expandable, i.e. not requiring chairs or lab equipment in a classroom.

During my second year of medical school near the time that we had to decide where to transfer I went to lunch at the Student Union. While there I heard one of the students discussing a friend one year ahead of us who had transferred to West Virginia Medical School. When he said "West Virginia" a special alertness was awakened above me like a light flash. I began to look into it as an option. Although I applied to two other schools I ended up there. West Virginia turned out to be an excellent school for me because it fit my special medical interests in important ways. They had an unusual and innovative psychiatry program and it was close to a research institute that led to my residency in holistic medicine.

Intuition can be used for the mundane as well as major decisions. Knowing who is on the phone when it rings is a common experience of many. At times I have found parking spots quickly just where needed and when in a bit of a hurry. At other times, led by a hunch, I have followed up on an article in a science magazine or even the newspaper that led to fascinating and very helpful information and relationships. These hints of knowing lead us to an invisible connection that extends beyond the senses. The flash of insight is a sign we are connected with the world around us in subtle ways. This connection can make it easier for us to cooperate with it, learn from it and extend ourselves further with it.

Learn to Separate Instinct From Intuition

Instinct is the reflex to what happens to us. It is an almost automatic response without thought or consideration based on habit and familiarity. Physically, instinct is the jerk of the elbow when we accidentally hit a nerve like the funny bone and automatically rub it to decrease the pain. Emotionally, instinct is the response to laugh at a funny story or counter criticism quickly. Mentally, instinct is the use of the mind to recall a story similar to the one we just heard. These reactions are instinct at work, not intuition or the higher mind with its creative capacity of a higher perspective.

There are many kinds of instinct of varying complexity such as self-preservation, personal ambition, sex, family, and the need to learn. Each of these has its lower and higher aspects and is variable in its influence over us. The goal is to cooperate with them when needed but also to understand their control over us. The higher goal is to be creative instead of reactive, to use intuition instead of instinct to interact with life's challenges and mobilize the best within us.

One of the most compelling instincts is self-preservation. It is a very useful drive that often prevents injury and illness. The body uses this reaction to warn us about spoiled food and to fight an infection. We use instinct whenever we eat. However instinct does not always take into account the health of the whole. It is often driven by only one part of who we are like the taste buds choosing to satisfy themselves instead of the body as a whole. Unfortunately instinct may help us indulge comfort more than change. Do you want to be comfortable or do you want to change? Intuition is a skill for innovation and change.

Personal ambition is a common instinct. In the early stages of a developing ego ambition is a necessary way that we motivate ourselves. It is a major impulse we use to learn how to extend and expand ourselves in whatever career or project chosen. Ambition helps us learn skills of finding a job, maintaining a job and developing a healthy relationship with authority. With ambition we learn how to initiate and deepen important relationships with those who can help us, teach us and love us. There are reasons to go beyond accumulating stuff and things, comforts and pleasures, and attention that is ego satisfying. Expecting some credit for tasks well done is one thing; demanding it or resenting others for not giving it is quite another. Intuition can enhance ambition but is also a means to go beyond it from the personal to the transpersonal.

Eventually the goal is for the higher self to dominate our agenda of action and motivation, not personal ambition. This usually means finding ways to serve others. It does not mean to deprive self, belittle self or jeopardize the future to help another. It means to have a high priority to be part of the solution for relieving the suffering of others, not to become part of the problem that adds to the suffering.

A strong instinct instead of intuition is especially prominent with sexual drive. This instinct is greater in some than others but must be confronted eventually. This is a powerful drive that is physically satisfying when met but is often only temporary. When controlled by personal desire more than concern for another it often leads to relationship difficulties and, too frequently, major discord and deep resentment. The sexual drive is meant to be expressed as part of a deepening relationship based on mutual devotion and dedication to another, not just self. It serves nature's laws of attraction and love which is fulfilled with giving and receiving. These laws also apply within self to how the lower and higher parts of ourselves are meant to grow and develop as well. Intuition can help guide the sexual impulse and the subtle energies of the relationships to which it leads.

Family and herd instinct naturally takes us beyond ourselves to our immediate and extended family. The benefits of family are immense and meant to be a major part of the launching pad for each of us. The positive elements of a healthy family include goodwill to all members, tolerance for differences and ready forgiveness for transgressions. A family spirit supports new beginnings in relationships, children, and career. It helps us with invaluable lessons in how life unfolds. The seeds of intuition are often planted in our family relationships because of the close bonds that connect our hearts and minds together.

The goal of the groups to which we belong is the purpose for which it lives and thrives. The challenges of family can be very daunting and at times traumatic. As the opportunities are taken and the conflicts confronted growth occurs, and we are slowly initiated into the larger groups of our community. These connections lead to larger problems, greater missions and the energies of them. As we learn how to identify, support or change the group to which we belong we extend our capacities for contributing to the larger whole. In the process we learn how to access greater strength for ourselves and the creative urges that drive us on. Intuition can guide this process of group involvement and a higher dimension of self-discovery.

The instinct to grow and learn is also a deep urge within us. When young it helps us to feed ourselves, protect ourselves and learn how to interact with others. Eventually we learn how to find a job, career or family that not only supports us but also makes life interesting. The use of intuition can save a great deal of pain and suffering during these times.

An essential ingredient of learning is the presence of curiosity. The more we have the faster and further we may find our lives unfolding. Its lowest level is noticing change in our immediate environment like a car accident or new scene of nature. The higher reaches of curiosity lead us to explore the wonderful landscapes of nature, art and music. Within ourselves the spirit of curiosity can lead us to be receptive to the higher life, its support, guidance, forgiveness and true delights. Our goal is to discern the ideal which means to find the best steps to take today in the use of our time and opportunities.

Intuition can be a reassuring tour guide as we pursue the string of experiences that unfold before us, pointing out warnings, insights and synchronicities.

What Is The Source of Intuition?

The source of intuition is within. What does that mean? Is it in the gut, the feeling department or in the air around us? It is often referred to as these but hopefully comes from the soul, the source of our life, the wisest part of who we are. The soul is the prime initiator of new ideas, new directions and the creative spark. The trigger may be an idea we read about in the newspaper, an event that happens in our lives, a word we see, a song we hear or a dream we have. But it may be the soul that is energizing it so that we pay attention. Particularly when it has a statement to make the soul will look for a way to motivate us to act or at least to ponder an option more carefully.

In some ways intuition is like a movie production. These require many players including the writer, producer, director, actors and support staff. The producer is usually the inspiration and motivator that sets all the others into action. The director helps choose the key staff, especially the actors, and then provides intelligent instruction, disciplined guidance and nurturing support. The actors are responsible for learning their roles, identifying with their characters major characteristics and serving the story.

The higher self, the soul, is the real source of new action. The source is like the writer, the fountain of inspiration who has a mission to make a statement. It attracts a producer, the personality, with an ambition to make a difference or contribute something worthwhile. The mission attracts a director as a dominant part of the personality with many internal actor options. Many of the actors arise from the mind and the heart, the feeling and experiencing center within. Our past is the source of most of our habits of expression drawn from the many experiences we have had since birth and maybe even before birth. The deeper we go in search of talent the more likely we'll find characters who represent distinct patterns of behavior that represent the best of who we are and have to offer. This is the role that intuition can invoke.

The Wizard of Oz provides a metaphor of how these parts works together. The Tin Man is the part of us who is weak in heart, initially timid and shy. He has the ability to feel a connection with people, to have friends and not be isolated from others. The Straw Man is missing a brain, the part of us that is naive, does not think too well and knows too little about who we are. He seems unable to make intelligent decisions or understand motives of unkind people or the self-serving parts of ourselves. And there is the Lion that represents the lack of strength when we need it, to speak up, to stand up for ourselves and to face obstacles until we overcome them. He is designed to have courage, initiative and strength when needed.

Dorothy is the striving to be the integrated personality with each of these different parts within her. The Straw Man, Tin Man and Lion represent her heart, mind and will. Each of these proceeds on the journey to realize their intended goals, to find greater expression of love, wisdom and courage. The soul is eager to work with whatever part will respond or most needs help at the time.

The skill of intuition helps us remember who we are, the purposes of our life and how to find their best expression. The hints and nudges are constantly awaiting only recognition to be awakened. Setting aside time and study to review the past and consider the future helps us be receptive to the guidance available. Choosing and allowing ourselves to be part of the action increases the chances to perfect our roles in the larger drama of which we are all a part. There are always a great number of rehearsals, trials and errors and ways to improve our performance. Intuition helps us find the patience and persistence we need to work with the source and express it fully.

Obstacles to Intuition

The most common obstacle is lack of interest, not knowing or caring enough to consider the fact that higher guidance is available. We are not trained to consider intuition as a skill of living and are much less likely to consider it because of that. However, many of us also become earth bound in recognizing only the physical world as real, the sensations of what we can see, hear, taste and touch. We miss the subtle hints and nudges of synchronicities and do not consciously consider intuition enough value to study and develop.

The real obstacles to successful uses of intuition are the excuses we use to distract, blame and complain. These will disconnect us from the missions we have and prevent our antenna from receiving the continual input we need to make each day new and worthwhile. When excuses outnumber solutions we are a long way from sources of inspiration.

Fears, doubts and worries are stop signs and roadblocks. They inhibit our ability to see what lies ahead by slowing our awareness of inner associations, memories and feelings. They decrease the number of contacts available and the richness that accompanies them. When negative obsessions take over we temporarily shut down and halt our input. At times such delays are useful if we take the time to identify the clutter of frustration and disappointment that has accumulated to organize it better. More often we feed our fears and worries by reminding ourselves how important they are instead of activating the solutions in front of us. When we overlook forgiveness of ourselves and others and the strengths we need to press on we obstruct the intuitive impulse of common sense.

Faith fatigue is a common obstacle. Lack of physical energy does impede us to some degree but fatigue of the heart and mind are far more debilitating. This usually occurs as a result of giving up too easily and lacking confidence in our ability to move ahead. Of course this is an excuse to sit back and wait for someone else to do the work. Such an attitude really exposes a faulty assumption that life is meant to be a relaxing comfortable journey that we are meant to enjoy life without much effort on our part. The reality is that it is up to us plot the course, drive the car and complete the mission. We each have several places to go and people to meet with a variety of routes and speed bumps on the way. The solution to fatigue is to find what is interesting on the road we travel. We need to take the risks to explore the landscape of options available and change course when necessary. On the way we learn how to use the tools of the heart and mind that includes an active imagination and intuition.

Extraordinary Uses of Intuition

Most dramatic uses of intuition are due to life threatening circumstances. When my sister was attending college she was over a thousand miles away.

One night I was awakened suddenly remembering only the words, "Help Rose." Two nights later I called to see how she was doing. When I related my experience there was a pause and she said, "Jim, you aren't going to believe this…" relating a very difficult time she was having with a boy friend at that exact time. There was a dispute and he shoved her causing intense fear for herself. Fortunately there was not further injury and the relationship ended soon after. But I was struck by how connected we were during this time of turmoil in spite of the distance. From this experience I learned to respond sooner to unusual calls for help.

Unfortunately most people do not pay attention to intuitive warnings. And when they do there is not a guarantee that events will change. In *The Gift of Healing* by Sally Rhine and Michael Schmicke they surveyed many people with intuitive premonitions. They found that half the time our interest in avoiding trouble pays off and damage is avoided. However, this means that half the time, even with warning, we are unable to avoid consequences of choice patterns set in motion.

The daughter of a close friend had a remarkable experience that helped her heal a difficult relationship. Her stepfather had been deteriorating in health and mood for several years. Disregard and obnoxious behavior for himself, his wife and her caused major distress. At a certain point she expressed herself strongly about how irresponsible he was, how difficult he was to live with and how hard it was making their life together. Over the next few days he deteriorated to the point of having to go to the hospital where he was diagnosed with congestive heart failure. Although he initially responded to intravenous medication he later expired in the hospital. She felt an intense remorse for what she had said in spite of knowing it was true.

Several weeks later on an airplane flight home she related the following event. "I was looking out the plane window and saw the 'green flash' at a very precise moment when the sun sets. [Her step-father] used to speak of that moment but I had never seen it. At that moment he was very clearly speaking to me in my head and apologizing for his selfish and hurtful behavior. I remember crying and forgiving him. It felt like a long moment but it happened in that instant. Afterwards I felt very peaceful and fully forgave him for his bad behavior."

Intuition can save our life. Only a few years ago the father of a good friend in high school wrote an autobiography. He was an unusually outgoing fellow seemingly always cheerful and enjoyable to see. He always had at least a few new funny stories to share and loved exchanging them with everyone he met. While his son and I were in college he became executive secretary to the governor of North Dakota where I was raised. Governor Link was re-elected and Woody retained his advisory relationship to the Governor for eight years altogether.

However in his book I learned for the first time of an event that happened during World War II. Because of his intelligence, active interest in people and fluency in French he rose quickly through the ranks. At one point he was in charge of a shipload of troops being transported from England to France right after D-Day. The night before departure he was in a bar chatting with Navy personnel. He was told that another ship was sailing that evening allowing him to arrive early to prepare the landing site for his men.

The next day while waiting for his ship to arrive he saw them begin to approach the shore from a few miles away. There was a large explosion and the ship began to sink, most likely hit by a German torpedo. As a result of his decision the night before he was in a position to offer more help than if he was with his men on board. He was able to mobilize rescue and his life was saved most likely for a very good reason. He had a great deal to offer others. His intuition to accept the offer to ship over the previous night saved his life and provided many more the opportunity to benefit from his intelligent love and wisdom.

Such guidance is most likely a planned event by those available to help us. Fortunately he was receptive to a creative opportunity and he acted on it. Being attentive to the possibility of new unplanned options is an important step in using intuition. Acting on it is the other essential ingredient.

Intuition can help us excel at our job. As a young woman my aunt had a job with a large insurance company. She was trained to enter the incoming checks into the up-to-date registry system. At the end of the day she had to balance the entries of the day. If her ledger numbers were not in balance, she would have to go over the entries until mistakes were identified. This could become very time-consuming and required her and several of the other clerks to stay hours after closing. Even then mistakes were not always found that day.

After a few long days and having to begin the next day behind she began to awaken at night with a memory of the entered mistakes. During the night she remembered rising out of her body, floating to the office and reviewing the entries of the day. The mistakes would be highlighted for her to notice and she would make a mental note of which ones they were. In the morning she would review the list and found that her nighttime visit was accurate. It reached the point that if she did not balance by the end of the day her immediate supervisor would say "Let Tress sleep on it" and out the door they would go.

When there is a need to know the higher mind is ready to help us with the tool of intuition. This is most likely the case far more than we realize. It is a matter of recognizing that the higher mind has the answer, knows what has happened and already has a solution.

Practical Steps That Awaken The Voice of Intuition

Intuition is a language that requires an increasing awareness of inner sounds, reactions and memories. Young parents of a newborn child soon learn the many sounds of their baby. Various grunts, gasps and cries all have different meanings. The fortunate child has parents who pay attention and are willing to learn and respond to the new language. In the same way we each have a language of memory flashes of old friends and events may be connections that are revealing an inner knowing and a true meaning of current concerns that is more reliable than our usual input of vision and hearing.

Here is a list of practical ways to improve our skills of intuitive perception:

1. Begin the day with at least a brief period of time that identifies the best within. Commune with the higher self however you understand that to be. Devote yourself to its purpose and plan for you at this time of your life. Know that its intention is for your highest good in spite of the suffering, loss or disappointments you now carry.

2. Review the day that just passed. What did you do well? What did you not do well? What did you overlook? What hints did you receive that helped you respond well? What hints did you receive but did not act on?
3. Ask for what strength you most need at this time with your current responsibilities and opportunities. Is it courage, resilience, persistence or patience? Is it forgiveness, tolerance, kindness and cheerfulness? Choose one for this day.
4. Consider the day before you. What are the key events most likely to occur? How would you like them to unfold? What qualities of mood and thought do you most want on your mind when these happen? Ask for help to remember what these are just before and during the events. Imagine a successful outcome with the events and people you are most likely to see this day.
5. Look for chances to reflect on what is happening during brief lulls in the day. Jot down or even discuss interesting observations, memories or possibilities that come to you during the day.
6. Be grateful for the guidance you receive however subtle whether directly from within or from someone else.
7. Continuously rededicate yourself to being of help, alert to the task at hand and the inner resources available. Ask for help, challenge what you receive and look for ways to express what seems to fit.

In these ways we can mobilize the power of intuition to better listen, learn and heal.

Chapter 16

Dreams Reveal Causes and Cures

Dream activity has been recorded since the beginning of time. The Bible has many references to dreams and dream interpreters, providing as many warnings against the use of dreams as for them. It also has several prominent events surrounding the use of dreams. The most well known is the one of Joseph, the son of Jacob. His ability to interpret the Pharaoh's dream not only freed him from prison but also established him as a major advisor, and most importantly, saved the lives of thousands from starvation including his own family.

In ancient Greece dreams were a prominent part of the healing approaches used at the Aesculapian Temples. Founded by Aesculapius around 1000 B.C., they provided care and healing for many for almost 1500 years. Diet, exercise, self-reflection and the use of emulating heroes and heroines were common recommendations for treatment. At times people were referred to the Oracles at Delphi, experts in the art of intuitive guidance and healing. At Delphi suggestions were also given to attend an Aesculapian Temple.

However the most dramatic healings occurred with dream incubation. Individuals were encouraged to invoke healing during the sleep state. This often resulted in a visit by a healing spirit who either radiated healing energy or gave advice in how to heal self. In any event, many healings of serious illness are recorded from such special visits.

A Healing Dream Project

During my residency in Holistic Medicine, I organized a dream incubation project. I invited patients with chronic sinusitis to join a dream workshop. We met once a week for two hours for eight weeks requesting a dream to help heal the sinus condition. Eight patients enrolled and attended most of the meetings. None of them had training in dream recall or interpretation. During the workshop everyone's ability to remember dreams improved, as did the ability to understand and learn from the dream state.

One participant was especially skilled at remembering her dreams. When she recounted a dream we were in for a twenty minute story. Near the end of the project she brought the most interesting dream. It was again a lengthy one. At one point, near the end of the dream, she recounted entering a small room, all white and unfurnished. Upon going through the doorway she saw a scorpion on the floor at which point a loud voice said, "That's why you have sinusitis." We went through the dream one piece at a time, finally coming to the scorpion. I asked her what a scorpion has to do with her life. She said, "It must be my husband, he's a Scorpio."

I began to ask about their relationship. We learned that they had been married eighteen years and that she began sinus problems seventeen years ago. I asked about their first year of marriage and if there had been any major concern or worry for her during that time. She said that there was but that she had never discussed it with him. I suggested that she look for a time the next week to bring it up, a time when they seemed especially close or at least very comfortable together.

The following week she reported that they had the discussion recommended and that she was satisfied with the answer given. Soon thereafter she began to notice improvement in the sinus congestion. Over the next few weeks she had complete resolution of her chronic sinusitis. One year later she was still doing quite well without sinus congestion recurrence.

It is apparent that her sinus condition was related to an unresolved issue with her husband. There was a congestion of apprehension that resulted in a physical congestion. She confronted the situation effectively, no longer fearful of the response of her husband. Her subconscious responded to her request for healing with a dream.

The body's ability to heal is quite remarkable. It is not as stuck or static as we may think, even for long-term chronic conditions. The energy is really more frozen at the emotional level than the physical. When we re-set how we feel we free up the energy to flow more freely. I do not think it is a matter of just wanting to be well that brings forth the healing. If so there would be many more reports of rapid healing than we hear. This woman healed herself because she worked through the frustration over the years in her marriage with her husband. The dream was a trigger for the final healing event. Although it appeared to be a sudden response most likely there had already been a concerted effort to be patient, forgiving, tolerant and loving. These energies coalesced in the conscious decision to confront the underlying problem through a dream and subsequent discussion with her husband.

A Warning Dream Can Be Healing

William Dement is one the pioneers of sleep medicine. As a psychiatrist he was by training interested in the sleep state. Early in his career he began to study the sleep state and helped to identify and clarify the role of the rapid eye movement (REM) stage. In his book on sleep disorders, *The Promise of Sleep*, he recounts this event in his life:

"One morning I awoke coughing and coughing until I began to see blood coming up. I was quite worried because I knew this could be a sign of lung cancer. I was a psychiatrist at the time and immediately called my physician friend who performed a chest x-ray. I watched the film develop and the radiologist put it on the film display stand. It was quite clear there was a large mass, very characteristic of severe lung cancer. I was aghast at the thought that I probably had only a short time to live. I became very distressed with the fact that I had developed a three-pack per day smoking habit knowing it was harmful. I could only groan deeply of the effect on my family and work that I would miss." Then he woke up from the dream.

He subsequently listened to the dream, stopped smoking and has lived well into his 80s with no lung cancer ever developing. Fortunately for him, his subconscious was strong enough to break through and show him the consequences of his unhealthy behavior. A very dedicated life can expand access to the healing energies we need through a dream.

Edgar Cayce says that we dream all major events before they happen. If this is so why do so many of us continue to get into so much trouble with disease, injuries and stupid mistakes? The simple answer is that we do not pay attention. The more complicated answer is that we do not want to change who we are and the habits we have. Do you want to be comfortable or do you want to change?

One woman came to our morning dream class with a question about a budding relationship. Although they were only recently acquainted he looked like a promising companion. He asked her to meet him in Paris for a potential trip together. I suggested that she ask for a dream to guide her decision of whether to join him or not.

Within a few days she brought a dream to the group. She was in Paris at night, winding her way through narrow streets not knowing where she was or how to find her way. In the dream she felt lost, worried and distressed. In exploring the dream with her it was obvious to us that the answer was clear. Her subconscious was showing her what it thought about this relationship, especially the pending trip that she was considering. She did not accept this suggestion and took the trip. I had occasion to see her several weeks later. She said she had a terrible time and regretted making the trip.

The subconscious can only present what is happening; the interpretation and meaning remain up to us. We can choose to see the obvious or ignore it until the signs are clearer. Dreams are a great avenue to mobilize healing power if we are willing to listen.

Healing A Repetitive Dream

Healing dreams can help us heal the heart and mind. At times certain fears are imbedded in the subconscious waiting for the proper sincere search for new ways to heal. A woman recalled a repetitive dream that she called the "ringing phone dream." She said that she had this dream usually when there was a great deal of stress in her life. The dreams began following an experience she had one night when her husband called her on the phone to announce that he wanted a divorce. This was a major surprise to her and became a depressing turning point in her life.

While at Meadowlark retreat center she made a major effort to learn about herself and make healthier changes in her life. Near the end of her two-week stay she had the ringing phone dream and, for the first time, was not afraid. This was a major sign of progress she was making and greater acceptance of who she was.

Repetitive dreams usually begin with a major emotional event of some kind. It may not always be felt that way at first and may be denied as important to protect ourselves from the pain. However in work with dreams it is often helpful to review preceding events and reactions. Healing occurs as we confront ourselves and the fears we harbor and the sense of weakness, inadequacy or stubbornness. As we do this we then mobilize the courage needed for healing. We discover that the darkness does not contain a monster, only our fear of one. What is missing is our strength to take a stand with ourselves and express who we are. We heal repetitive dreams by confronting the current and past issues to which they may be connected.

Exposing The Inner Critic Can Be Healing

Dreams often reflect current concerns and worries. One man had the following dream: "I am in a kitchen cooking a meal. A friend tastes it and makes an expression of displeasure. I say, 'It's not good.' She shakes her head. I tell her, 'Jim told me to fix the meal.'"

He was a screenwriter for a TV show. In trying to meet a deadline he submitted a re-write with which he was not satisfied. After this dream he realized he had to do another re-write, which he did. He used the critical feedback and made the proper adjustment.

If we need honest assessment we need look no further than our own inner critic present in a dream. A middle-aged man reported the following dream to me: "I'm in a large mansion with many, many rooms and many,

many people. It is a wonderful atmosphere. There are two albinos smoking hash. People begin to move outside. I see a woman but have little contact with her. Another woman says, 'You aren't wanted. You make things worse. She doesn't want you.' The words boom out 'You have a powerful influence on others. When you criticize them you add to their problem.'"

He admitted to making quick judgments about people and recalled recently seeing an overweight woman. His initial reaction was that all she needed was some discipline. Then he remembered the dream. He learned that just his negative impressions of others had a potential harmful effect on them and himself. He valued the insight. His habit of being quick to criticize was exposed in the dream and he chose to use it to make the changes necessary.

The goal is to honor the inner critic but not put it in charge. Integrity is a strength that we all need in full amount. Most of us don't have enough. The inner critic needs to be an ally in the effort. However, some of us have a tendency to give too much authority to the inner critic and thereby belittle ourselves and others in the process. Such a reaction will cause us to inhibit ourselves and limit our ability to interact with others and what they have to offer us.

Dreams are like a mirror of our inner life, our energy memory storage of how we think and feel. If we are willing to be honest with ourselves dreams can be an excellent way to review what to change and how. It is very much like watching a movie of ourselves. We see how we react to life's events and the reasons to change who we are. With discernment and determination we can recreate ourselves into more than who we've been and closer to who we will become.

The Prayer of St. Francis can be an excellent guideline for finding the right sense of self toward which we aspire in our lives and in our dreams.

Lord, make me an instrument of your peace.
Where there is hatred, let me sow love.
Where there is injury, pardon.
Where there is doubt, faith.

Where there is despair, hope.
Where there is darkness, light.
Where there is sadness, joy.

O Divine Master,
grant that I may not so much seek to be consoled, as to console;
to be understood, as to understand;
to be loved, as to love.
For it is in giving that we receive.
It is in pardoning that we are pardoned,
and it is in dying that we are born to Eternal Life.

St. Francis himself had a dream encouraging him to start an order of monks. He went to Rome to request an official designation. The Pope participated in refusing the request and then had a dream. In the dream the Church, the Catholic Church, was falling apart. He saw one man with the Church on his back. It was Francis. He woke up and re-established contact with Francis, granting him the support he wanted. The Pope's initial criticism of Francis was exposed in a dream. Fortunately he paid attention to his higher conscience and rose above the critical self. The fact that Francis continues to inspire many almost 1,000 years later is the evidence that Pope Innocent III did the right thing, and that dreams can mobilize healing power.

Incubating A Healing Dream

We can get an answer to a question from a dream. At one point I was seeking direction how to be more effective with the patients that I see. I was not bored but I had the sense that I could be more effective with my patients than I was. One morning I woke with a dream. The dream was of me walking on the cliff overlooking the ocean. I saw an isthmus jutting into the water for quite a distance like a long pier. Just as I passed the isthmus continuing to follow the cliff I turned to look back onto the water. I noticed a shimmering light coming out of the water and then awoke.

A few weeks later I was leafing through a medical journal. I was struck when seeing an ad with the exact image of the shimmering light I saw in the dream. It was the picture of the tail of a whale just coming out of the water, creating a shimmering effect as the water ran off the tail. The caption underneath the ad was "A balance of gentleness and power." The message was the answer to the question.

The message to me was to look for ways to add power to my purpose in treating my patients. This was the response to my inner urge to do better from my higher self. I am sure I had seen the ad before but it did not register until I was consciously seeking insight how to do better. This insight continues to lead me to look for and find power within myself and those I see, especially the ones with difficult conditions that are hard to treat. It was very reassuring to ponder. In some way the insight helped me mobilize a greater sense of service that made a difference.

Jack Canfield is the co-author and founder of *Chicken Soup for the Soul.* When he had written the first book of the series he had difficulty finding the title. One morning he awoke from a dream. He was at his mother's kitchen table being served chicken soup. He awoke with the title on the tip of his tongue.

Dreams can be a way to mobilize healing power that affects millions of people.

Incubating a dream for healing can work. A few simple steps can invoke the help we need:

1. Choose one condition of which to ask for healing or direction.
2. Write out the events that have happened with this condition and why healing or direction is needed.
3. Ask a direct simple question about the condition; e.g. how did I contribute to this problem, in what way do I obstruct healing, what do I most need to forgive within myself or what do I most need to express to heal this problem?
4. Write out the question and place it with paper and pen by the bedside.
5. Ask for help in remembering dreams pertaining to this question.

6. Be willing to use whatever is remembered.
7. Work with whatever dreams or fragments of dreams are recalled looking for where the images, thoughts, feelings, and memories may lead.
8. Ask for help from a friend, mentor, counselor and higher self as needed.

Chapter 17

The Role of Healers in Self-Healing

My first study of extraordinary healing came with reading about Edgar Cayce. Early in his life certain events occurred that triggered a deep response within him, revealing an immense intuitive capacity to see the subtle energy patterns of people's illnesses and circumstances. As he successfully diagnosed and recommended certain treatments for seemingly incurable conditions, his reputation expanded. Near the end of his life he had given "readings" for about 12,000 people with a wide variety of medical diseases, with many innovative treatments some of which were not discovered by mainstream medicine for over fifty years. In the mid 1970s the New England Journal of Medicine had an article referring to him as the father of holistic medicine.

Mr. Cayce was especially known for the succinct phrase that "The spirit is the source, mind the builder and the body the result." This is a powerful philosophical focus that describes how we create chasms in our life and can find our way out. It describes the cause of much disease and how to heal from it. We are each a center of creative energy born with a creative fire enabling us to build or destroy. The primary goal is to align with our Spirit and compel ourselves to serve its agenda above all. This is how we mobilize our own power for healing.

James L. Kwako, M.D.

One of the most dramatic healings that came through Mr. Cayce was among the first on which he was consulted. It was for a six year old, Anne Dietrich, the daughter of a professor and superintendent of schools in Hopkinsville, KY. When a toddler, probably just over one year old, she had diphtheria that caused brain damage, convulsions and subsequent lack of physical and mental development. She was taken to many specialists who said that she would die soon. Edgar said her condition was NOT directly related to diphtheria, but that she had received an injury to the spine prior to the infection. The diphtheria caused a breakdown in the injured spine tissues resulting in scar tissue formation. Cayce recommended spinal adjustments to loosen the area. "Then nature will take its course. She will recover," he said in trance. The parents followed his instructions with the help of an osteopath and repeat readings to assess guidelines for spinal adjustments. Within three weeks she could sit up and cut out pictures with a scissors. Within three months she was a normal child. She graduated from college at the top of her class.

Mr. Cayce talked about energy systems of the body that are not covered in medical school. Although he was quite aware of the usual organ function, he saw an interaction that was much more dynamic from organ to organ and from mind to body. The information that came through him was so compelling it led me to doing a residency in Holistic Medicine at the Cayce Research Clinic.

During this residency program I heard about and then met a woman with scleroderma. This is an unusual connective tissue disorder that results in hardening of the skin, especially of the hands. The ends of the fingers actually become crystallized, resulting in loss of sensation and subsequent loss of use. Modern medicine still has little to offer. However, Cayce had given suggestions to several individuals with this condition, some of whom responded quite favorably.

The woman I met at the clinic had a documented diagnosis of scleroderma. It had been progressing for several years until she became a patient there. Over a period of several months of applying the suggestions recommended by Cayce to others with such a condition she began to improve. After a few years she was completely well except for small signs of hardened skin at the very tips of her fingers. There were no longer any intestinal symptoms, fatigue or other systemic complications common to scleroderma.

My mother-in-law was also diagnosed with scleroderma. When told that nothing more could be done she asked for my help in applying the Cayce suggestions. She began to follow a healthier diet, stretch on a daily basis, began to use a special, very low current electrical device and work on improving her mood and mind. After several months she began to notice definite signs of improvement. Two years later she was proclaimed by her doctor to be free of scleroderma.

The best summary of Mr. Cayce's remarkable career is well recorded in *Edgar Cayce: An American Prophet* by Sidney Kirkpatrick.

Olga Worrall

The most effective healer I have had a chance to know and study with is Olga Worrall. She was born with the gift of healing, and, typical of great individuals, her experiences began early. Friends, family and especially her mother responded to her loving presence and laying-on-of-hands when ill or in pain. She also married a healer, Ambrose Worrall, an English immigrant. Together they were a formidable team. By the time I met Olga her husband had passed on. I attended one of the many classes she taught about healing. She was often cheerful about her life but serious about healing. A few miraculous healings occurred, and she would say, just to let us know what is possible, that God is present. She had a deep regard for the process of healing and those who were part of "the team," i.e. spirits helping from the other side. She especially delighted in showing pictures of spirits present during the healing process. The figures were easy to see and clearly definable.

She and her husband's explanations for how healing occurs are instructive. There is a well-developed inner transformer in the healer, closely connected to the soul of the healer. This is a built-in, born-with device, part of the subtle energy field of the healer. That does not mean that others cannot heal but that dramatic changes are less likely. The transformer adjusts the energy current needed to the frequency that can be received by the patient. The healer must also be a transformer matching the energy source of the patient to allow the healing current to have the proper effect. The healing current utilizes the nervous system of the patient. The Worralls describe healing as a rearrangement of the micro particles, of which all things are composed, about which we continue to learn more and more and have much further to go.

"Calmness, peace, gentleness and patience" are effective conditions for healing. These need to be present to some degree in the patient for there to be connection channels to receive the healing energy and to prevent static for the effective flow of vital energy.

The main reason why healing occurs is that the healing channel is open for God to do what can be done. "I am only a channel, an instrument of Higher Power," Olga would say often. If healing does not occur, the patient is not ready, the healer is not adaptable to the patient or a number of other possibilities may prevent it.

My older brother met Olga at the second annual meeting of the American Holistic Medical Association. He asked for help with his chronic, intermittent migraine headache condition. The headache disappeared with the treatment though they did return from time to time thereafter.

Olga occasionally visited the Pain Clinic where I was working. On one particular occasion, Dr. Shealy was hosting an NBC film crew for a special piece on people with unusual abilities. It was called "Psychic Phenomena--Exploring the Unknown," and Olga was the featured healer. One patient on whom she worked was a 46-year-old truck driver with chronic low back pain. He had two major operations for relief and was attending our clinic. He had decreased his medication to some degree but was still in a great deal of pain by the time of this treatment. Olga was in another room about fifty feet away. At a signal from her the healing began and proceeded for 5-10 minutes. The patient initially had a body shake, seemed to tighten briefly, then relaxed comfortably. After the treatment he said, "That felt great." He was pain-free for several weeks after which some of the pain returned.

The most dramatic success was a construction worker with whom she worked. He came to the pain clinic because of bladder cancer. It was invasive throughout much of the bladder and surrounding area. He was told that surgery could be done but that it would be very extensive, not a guarantee of cure and that he would lose all sexual capacity. He was recently married and was not interested in surgery. He went to Olga's healing clinic in Baltimore. Six week later he called to say that he had just returned from a visit to his urologist. His doctor said that he could not believe that the tumor was essentially gone, there were only two small areas of inflammation left, and they did not look like cancer. The patient was thrilled with the results.

When I asked him if I could share his story he said, yes, and "tell them that if all this crazy stuff can work for this dumb bastard, it can work for anyone." It is worth emphasizing that he was well motivated to be with his new wife, and he was willing to expose himself to totally new ways of thinking.

A Philippine Healer

Another visitor to the clinic for the NBC special was a healer from the Philippines. He was a young man, in his thirties, dressed in a short-sleeved white shirt and pants. He was pleasant, kind and quiet. He spoke English well though he had to be encouraged to describe what he did. He worked on five patients over a two-day period. I observed him work on most of the patients. I was quite aware of the history of their chronic pain problems and had examined each of them prior to the treatment with him. During the treatments he worked on different parts of their bodies. They were usually lying on their back with arms and hands at the sides. He would use his hands that seemed to penetrate the abdomen during which time red fluid appeared with small pieces of nonspecific tissue. At no time did it appear to me that he was inside the abdomen like I have seen in surgical operations where organs are visible. He worked for 15-20 minutes on each one.

At the end of each treatment, it was clear that two of the six were sure that he was helpful and that they had complete pain relief. I contacted each of them one month and six months later. At one month, the same two said they were still somewhat better from the treatments, though pain had returned to some degree. However at six months none of them were willing to say the treatment had been helpful. He may well have been more successful in his own culture. He did say that it is common knowledge that the appearance of blood-like tissue is materialized "for the belief of the patient." Such an experience may not be compelling enough for many in this country, at least for long term healing.

Negative Healing Effects

I have also had negative experiences with healers. At Meadowlark we had a woman guest who was also a healer. She attended the program for herself and found it to be quite helpful. Following several discussions with the administrator she was invited to participate as a consulting staff member. She taught classes, counseled guests and at times did healing. Many spoke highly of her benefits to them. However there was one guest who had a diagnosis of a type of lymphoma. After her healing session the healer told the patient that the cancer was gone, that she was well. The guest returned at another time and seemed well. However two years later she was found to have a recurrence of the lymphoma. The healer did visit her at her home city to help further. I did not hear the outcome.

This incident made it clear to me that no healer should proclaim a cure they cannot substantiate. The field of medicine is very careful about stating that a condition has been cured or healed when only the symptoms have improved or even disappeared. Healing can occur physically without trace of disease and yet with the pattern of consciousness of disease still present. The real goal of healing is to cure the consciousness of disease by replacing it with an ideal presence of life.

Healing is a complicated process especially for serious or chronic conditions. It involves much more than the physical body that we inhabit. The bodies of feeling, mind and memory are much more complex than the physical body's collection of organs and cells. There is much we do not know and must still explore. At times healings do occur, but usually not unless there is an evident deep sense of reverence and trust in a divine, higher power. "Thy will be done" not mine, is a common determining factor in mobilizing the presence of life.

Soon after I moved to Santa Barbara, I was asked to see a home-bound patient with advanced breast cancer. It seemed to me that she was dying from cancer metastases. She was intent on overcoming it and was asking for any aid that I could give her. We talked about various options, and she did her best to follow through with them. She also had requested the aid of a Shaman, a native American healer. When asked what the healer told her about the problem, she said "that tissue on the surface that was bleeding was dead cancer cells that the body was eliminating." He was quite sure the cancer was dying, but I was not. The patient died a few months later.

It is possible the healer prolonged her life a bit more, but I am more concerned that he misled her into thinking that she was healing when in fact she was not. Her final few months might have been better used by preparing for her demise, putting her life in order and gracefully accepting the immanent change that was occurring. The triggering event of cancer for her was a deeply disappointing relationship with which I'm sure she made progress.

Healing the cause of the problem should always be the ultimate goal, not healing the physical body. The real cause usually resides in the emotional or mental body rather than the physical. We often can identify what that is and must invoke the power of the healing presence to heal it. To focus mainly on the physical condition and expecting physical changes of the apparent illness is often missing the mark and will not sufficiently mobilize effective healing energy.

Malcolm Smith

Within the past few years I have learned about another healer, Malcolm Smith. He is an Englishman who was born in the coal mining area of England where he left school at age 15 to follow his father into the mines. Although first appearing in childhood, he did not turn to healing until the age of 33, when a series of events again unmasked this ability. He pursued training and study that led to increasing opportunities for healing, primarily through the support of the Edgar Cayce organization. He mainly does laying-on-of-hands but also distant healing.

The stories of healings about him are compelling, including a wide range of pain conditions, severe heart disease and metastatic cancer, including melanoma. About 80% of his patients improve in some way. Although many experience improvements, major changes do not occur quickly and most require 3-4 sessions.

Although he does not elaborate on the explanations of the healing process and what happens through him, he does clearly state that "Healers don't heal, God does the healing." He summarizes his thoughts on healing by stating that miracles do happen and symptoms can be relieved, but it is the cause that must be healed. The soul must by touched.

One of my patients had the following comments to say about his contact with Malcolm. "Over the last three weeks I have had some nasty seasonal allergies with a very sore and scratchy throat, puffy eyes and sinus pain. I was talking Allegra and Claritin and it was not helping at all. I get this every late May and all of June but this year was more extreme, and I was having a tough go of it and was holding on for early July when things always get better. Last Tuesday morning when Malcolm was here I had him do his regular healing on me, mostly for my gut as usual. I noticed nothing during the healing session. However as the day wore on I felt worse and worse. By evening I had a 103 fever with a headache and light nausea. I went to bed at 8 PM and woke up the next day feeling better. I drove Malcolm back to Wilma's and noticed that as the day went on the fever went away and I felt pretty good.

"This feeling good has continued and it is now nine days later. However, what I just realized today was that I have had no allergies after I had the fever of eight days ago, on the day Malcolm did the healing service. I am allergy-free and have not taken any meds. This is a first for me and I cannot attribute it to anything but the fever and Malcolm's treatment. Now did the treatment cause the fever and did that burn out the allergies? I have no clue. But I can say with confidence that I am allergy-free for now and I am surprised to say the least."

Other reports of healing were experienced by friends, family and myself. The above person's wife had an eye ailment that was continuously annoying and ophthalmologists were unable to help. In one session the irritation was gone and did not return. My mother-in-law began having chest pain that I diagnosed as angina heart pain. Within three sessions the pain was gone and she did not die of a heart attack, surviving for several more years. I began having right hip pain several years ago, a mild form of osteoarthritis. After three sessions it was gone and has not reappeared.

How To Choose A Healer?

Choosing a healer is like choosing a good friend. It usually does not happen suddenly, although some relationships advance more rapidly than others. These guidelines may be helpful:

1. Ask questions from whomever you first hear about the healer. What happens? What changes have you noticed? How were you treated as a person and a patient? The first contact may be sufficient in deciding whether to pursue a consultation.
2. Review whatever information is available. If a book is written and the matter is not urgent, read it carefully looking for how the story unfolds. Stories of healing should unfold naturally, not artificially or overly exaggerated. There should be honest accounts of difficulties and how they are overcome that are similar to others who struggle. Even excellent healers need to learn about the process and are willing to share how it unfolded.
3. Prices should be reasonable, especially if there is financial strain. A patient of mine who is not wealthy recently agreed to a telephone appointment with a popular psychic who charged $750 for 15 minutes. My patient was quite disappointed and properly disgusted with herself for pursuing the appointment. Olga and Ambrose refused to take any payment for their services that they saw as a gift from God.

In these days some fee is appropriate. Most genuine healers are very generous with their time and talent.

4. When setting up the appointment it is worth noticing the ease or difficulty, the interest or disinterest of those involved. To whom the healer attributes results is always a worthy question (it is not self). Look for clues as to the nature and depth of the healer. It is not necessary for the healer to know how or why healing occurs though some knowledge should be present.
5. It is especially helpful to prepare yourself physically and psychologically. Being rested, calm and arriving on time is respectful and necessary. Having thoughtful questions helps prepare the mind and body to be receptive to whatever healing may occur. Even rehearsing the encounter and asking for insight and guidance facilitates the healing process and opportunity.
6. Reviewing why healing is requested invokes a sense of responsibility. Some thought should be given as to how your life will be improved for the benefit of others with whatever healing is received.
7. These guidelines are very similar to those needed in seeing a doctor, a counselor, minister or rabbi for advice and counsel. Reasonable expectations are always necessary as life usually moves forward in decency and order. Whatever occurs beyond this is wonderful and worth deep gratitude. It is a higher power that guides the process. If more is to be learned before healing occurs, so be it. Be eager to learn it. Healing at the level most needed will arrive at some point in time.
8. Be grateful for any benefit gained to the healer and to the higher self within that recognized and pursued the opportunity presented.

Healers can mobilize healing power directly to us by their presence. In addition, many serve an excellent example of kindness, compassion, acceptance and understanding. A healer can become a role model for how to heal ourselves. We can repeat the experience in a morning meditation on a daily basis for a period of time. Such a practice can help us invoke our own healing power for our unique needs.

Chapter 18

How to Assemble a Team of Professional Practitioners

Soon after I finished medical training I attended a seminar on Hypnosis, Autogenics and Healing. The speaker was a neurosurgeon, Norm Shealy, who had recently started the comprehensive chronic pain treatment center at which I would later work. The first day of the seminar he offered to chat after dinner with anyone interested. There were maybe five of us. One fellow, David Harris, was from San Diego. He was very enthused about a more holistic, integrative approach to healing. He was quite sure this would be an area of great interest to the public and the medical field. Norm asked me what I thought and my first reaction was skeptical, as was his. I was hopeful but didn't see it happening soon. But we were both wrong.

David went on to form The Mandala Society. They organized a set of annual meetings for the next 10 years that helped to pioneer what became known as Holistic Medicine. The meetings brought together many experts in science, medicine and healing. The meetings were highly successful for many years, attracting people from around the U.S. and many other countries.

Within a few years Norm began to meet with a few other physicians very dedicated to the larger field of healing. With their help and support he began the American Holistic Medical Association, an organization of physicians and osteopaths dedicated to the principles of healing. The mission statement of the AHMA was to declare the nature of man as body, mind and spirit. Disease is an imbalance in one or more of these as well as their relationship with society and the environment. Healing occurs when these are brought into balance.

The role of the practitioner is to facilitate the work that must be done to improve the lifestyle and major relationships. The lifestyle changes often needed address the body, heart and mind. The physical body needs include establishing a healthy diet, exercise routine and productive activities. The heart requires learning about the emotional body; i.e. what are the common expressions that are unhealthy, which feelings are healthy and how to expand the use of them. The mind becomes healthy by using it to learn new skills, be informed about the needs of the community in which we live and find ways to be helpful to the people with whom we associate. The indwelling spirit helps us access the higher nature of ourselves and integrate it into our daily lives.

Holistic medicine appealed to many when it was first presented. However it was also not embraced by the medical field because of being too inclusive of a wide range of new and not easily verified, nonphysical approaches. In the last several years holistic medicine has evolved into alternative and then complementary care, the latter term promoted by like-minded British practitioners. These terms became subsumed into integrative medicine that is embraced by the medical field and is now found in most major medical centers in the country.

The annual meetings of the AHMA drew participants from all major fields of medicine. All the specialties were represented as well as most of the health fields of nurses, chiropractors, acupuncturists, naturopaths and others. While each of these groups has its own national and local organizations and gatherings, for the first time a holistic perspective was being added. Soon after the AHMA was formed a group of nurses began the AHNA that, along with the AHMA, continues to grow slowly but consistently. The American Holistic Medical Institute provides a specialty exam and credential in Holistic Medicine. In 2013 the new specialty of Integrative Medicine was born and is by the now recognized by the American Medical Association.

The primary emphasis in integrative medicine is in teaching healthy lifestyle living, especially good nutrition, diet and the use of supplements. There are many scientific studies supporting the use of these, and the number of studies reported each year continues to rise. Some studies are negative and not supportive of certain remedies under certain conditions. Because of the complexity of designing studies that are precise and replicable, one or even many studies of a given supplement are not enough to finalize value or discredit its use. Fortunately growing interest in the medical community is inspiring further research that is necessary to define parameters of use of the growing number of substances found in nature that may be of value.

Conventional medicine has its own problems verifying the value of medications and procedures. Even after many expensive studies and approval for the public, many medications are found to have serious adverse effects resulting in later withdrawal. The contention of integrative medicine practitioners is that natural, safer and less expensive remedies may be worth trying far more often to the benefit of many patients especially those with chronic disease.

The most important contribution of integrative medicine to conventional medicine is the emphasis on the role of the mind in disease. Medical studies have shown a vast number of ways that stress contributes to the onset and at times the cause of many conditions. The most obvious stressors are injuries, illness and surgery. Less obvious fears, doubts, and worries that are sustained over long periods of time often lead to a wide range of diseases.

Integrative medicine encourages a closer look at how our attitudes and reactions to life's circumstances contribute to the onset and the treatment of many illnesses. It is very reassuring to many to know how turning points of inner turmoil are part of the sequence of vulnerability. Most people know this intuitively but need professional support to pursue a fuller recognition of the impact of inner attitudes and psychological responses.

Integrative medicine practitioners are more likely to explore the role of the mind and thereby suggest psychological interventions. Appropriate counseling may be indicated as well as psychotropic medication. However there is also a growing number of innovative ways to use the mind to heal the body. The range of options should include relaxation training, biofeedback, neurofeedback, hypnosis, visualization, meditation, positive psychology, medical intuition and laying-on-of-hands healers.

The most common referrals by doctors of integrative medicine are to practitioners of chiropractic, massage, nutrition, acupuncture and homeopathy. Practitioners of these fields of healing are also more likely to be integrative in their approach, which means they are more likely to discuss the values of nutrition, supplements and other alternative approaches. The organizations most able to refer integrative practitioners are the American Holistic Medical Association, the American Holistic Nurses Association, Institute for Functional Medicine, the Institute of Integrative Medicine and the American College for the Advancement of Medicine.

Chiropractic and Osteopathic Spinal Adjustment

I first became involved in non-conventional medicine when in college. I injured my back in an athletic event and went to see a chiropractor. He was helpful and I became aware of the rationale behind the field. When I asked the advice of an orthopedic surgeon about chiropractic he was quite dismissive and critical. When I persisted in knowing the value of chiropractic, he told me he had a full practice and that I could go where I choose.

I discussed some of the principles of chiropractic in medical school. It was interesting to me to think of how an abnormality in one part of the body will cause trouble elsewhere. I was intrigued by this idea when studying anatomy and basic physiology. One day we were called together to meet with the dean of the school. No one knew why we were meeting since it was not a planned event. When we had gathered, the dean said there was talk about chiropractic among the students and that this was of great concern. He said that it was totally unscientific and not to be pursued.

The one who was discussing chiropractic was me, no one else. I was surprised there would be such a negative reaction. The threat to my medical career was clear, and I learned to be careful after that. However, my interest in it continued. The more I read and met with chiropractors, the more convinced I became of their capacity to help patients with a wide variety of ailments, especially spinal pain conditions. Fortunately times have changed, in part triggered by a successful lawsuit won by the Chiropractic organizations against the AMA. The main factor was a growing sense that people were getting better, pain was being relieved and physicians who knew of the benefits were speaking up. In addition there has been a growing number of studies clearly showing the value of chiropractic treatments.

Chiropractors are primarily trained to treat people with back pain and other musculoskeletal conditions. In conjunction with UCLA,, Rand Corporation sponsored research reviews of the benefits of chiropractic. They concluded that it especially works for those with acute low back pain but were inconclusive in the relief of chronic back pain. Like with many practitioners and physicians I have found that some are more skilled than others, and in some ways have more to offer. I have had several patients over the years who have responded very well to chiropractic adjustments. Many people use them for prevention as well as treatment, very successfully.

The function of the chiropractic adjustment is to readjust subluxations of the spine. These are misalignments that cause surrounding tissue swelling, pain and pressure on the nerves extending from the spine. Gross and subtle pressures can overexcite or inhibit normal nerve function leading to not only pain conditions but possibly organ function as well.

In non-back related problems there is less likely to be improvements, although there are many stories of success. One of the most dramatic conditions I have heard involved an individual with serious psychological problems. He was accused of serious physical abuse of his wife and children. Edgar Cayce related it to an injury to the spine and gave suggestions for the adjustments needed to reverse the problem. In spite of being in a psychiatric facility at the time, adjustments were allowed and resulted in a complete resolution of the disease and return to normal life of the individual.

Complications from chiropractic adjustments do occur. I do not see them often but have read and seen patients who have had fractured ribs from over-adjusting the spine, worsening of a pain condition and, at times, delayed use of better medical treatment.

Osteopathic Physicians also adjust the spine. The founder of osteopathy, A. T. Still, began teaching principles of osteopathy in 1874, approximately 20 years before D. D. Palmer founded chiropractic. Mr. Still emphasized natural laws of healing and the need to follow nature to promote healing. He also taught spinal adjustment techniques, mainly for musculoskeletal conditions. Generally speaking osteopaths adjust the spine in gentler ways than chiropractors. There are many techniques that have been developed over time, remarkably helpful for a wide range of conditions. The approach should definitely be used especially when other approaches have not worked. Highly skilled professionals in each group are quite effective and sensitive to the needs of the individual patient.

Osteopaths have the same basic science and clinical training as physicians. Most practice primary care medicine. Many specialize in one of the subspecialties of medicine though fewer than medical students. The difference in the training of osteopaths is the emphasis on spinal adjustments and a philosophy of healing, neither of which is taught in medical schools. They are also trained to do cranial-sacral adjustments used for a variety of musculoskeletal conditions especially in the head. Their philosophy of healing is based on observing and following nature, that disease is understandable and part of the orderly process of life. They are taught to respect the life within each person and all they bring to bear when presenting as a patient.

In 1954 Goeff Maitland began teaching spinal adjustment to physiotherapists. He developed expertise in gentle spinal adjustment. His skill, studies and articles have stirred a growing interest in the field of Physical Therapy toward tissue adjustment. At the pain clinic I had the chance to meet one of the well- trained physical therapists who uses this approach. He demonstrated the full use of the technique. It is gentle spinal adjustment and thus very unlikely to cause the rare but potentially serious adverse effects from more aggressive approaches.

Massage Is Rubbing People The Right Way

Massage is one of the most used forms of body therapy medicine. I first learned about therapeutic massage from Harold J. Reilly, a physiotherapist from New York City. He was active for over 60 years and tried retiring several times, each time returning to the work he loved. His definition of massage is simply rubbing people the right way. I became aware of him through the Edgar Cayce association. Mr. Cayce referred many people to him over his years of active work, considering him the best masseur in the upper Northeast.

The great American physician, William Osler, wrote a medical textbook that was in great use in the late 1800s and early 1900s. Under the section entitled "Lumbago," the term for chronic low back pain, he said that no cure was necessary because massage was so effective in most cases of it. In the right hands it is very effective. Many of my patients with acute and chronic back pain improve rapidly with comprehensive massage therapy.

Although physical therapists are officially trained to perform therapeutic massage, very few of them consider it a worthwhile and effective method. I think it is because modalities and therapeutic exercise has superseded the emphasis of massage in physical therapy school. For most conditions of chronic low back and neck pain I usually refer my patients to physical therapists who have expertise in massage. I want a therapist who believes in it, is trained to do it well and is effective. At times there are dramatic improvements and only occasionally are people made worse.

Adverse effects of massage occur mainly in the elderly due to being very sensitive to hard pressure. If overdone, the sensitive tissues become irritated, inflamed and swollen, increasing the lymph congestion instead of releasing it. To avoid this from happening I often encourage people to ask for what they need and provide feedback quickly if uncomfortable in any way. Sometimes discomfort is needed for a healing massage, at other times it is detrimental. The art of massage is knowing the difference.

Most deep tissue massage works by mobilizing vein and lymph tissue. These vessels are on the surface and the undersurface of the arms, legs, neck, back, chest and abdomen. The lymph tissue consists of cell debris, used chemicals and immune cell activity. The immune system is designed to fight infection, much of which occurs on the surface of the body. When infection is occurring regional lymph nodes increase their activity and often increase in size until the infection is under control. Although its vessels are small and the fluid moves slowly it can be increased with massage. Some therapists are trained in lymphatic drainage because of its therapeutic effects. Such treatments may improve lymph flow and decrease fluid accumulation. The stimulation of nerve endings and circulation increases immune activity and at times has a major benefit.

Besides providing therapeutic massage some therapists also develop the capacity to sense the subtle energy of the body. This is called the etheric body. This is the template for the physical body, and it has been studied by many individuals at great length. The etheric body extends 1-2 inches from the physical body and interpenetrates with it. It provides the energy and pattern for the physical organs and their function. Those who become familiar with it are aware of normal energy activity and obstructed or discordant circulating flow. At times their therapeutic efforts can make a difference in the finer energy body that is noticeable and endurable.

Massage treatment often leads to discussions of personal concerns. A good therapist will not only provide physical relief but a good ear and, at times, good advice as well. Some therapists are especially helpful in pointing out common sense views of handling current stress or at least refer people to those who can provide the psychological support needed.

Acupuncture Is Needling People The Right Way

Acupuncture is the ancient art of using fine needles to treat a wide range of diseases. Originating in China over 5000 years ago, it has had a resurgence of research and interest in the last 40 years. The end of the Cultural Revolution re-established a certain degree of stability for expanded study and teaching in China. President Nixon's historic visit to China in 1970 opened the door for Western medicine to become informed about and participate in the uses of acupuncture.

A great deal of study had accumulated prior to the recent past although references were difficult to find and translate. The current interest in acupuncture was reawakened over 80 years ago in France. A curious and courageous group of physicians discovered a treasure trove of records compiled by Catholic Jesuit priests over 500 years ago. The priests had visited China soon after the breakthrough visits by Marco Polo in the 14th century. Astute observers that they were, they compiled great detail about the practice of acupuncture, most likely from masters of the craft. A group of French physicians carefully studied the Jesuits' writings.

Joe Helms, M.D. became a student of the French acupuncture study group and helped bring it to the United States. After establishing a successful practice of acupuncture, Dr. Helms began to teach it to interested physicians, leading to the first physician acupuncture class in the U.S. at UCLA. Over 1,000 physicians have been trained by him and his team since 1985. Due to his efforts many medical centers and the military now incorporate acupuncture as standard treatment for a wide variety of medical conditions especially acute and chronic pain.

My first experience with doing acupuncture was with Dr. Shealy. He taught me the basic principles of needling and encouraged me to use it when I was working at the Pain Clinic, an ideal site for learning and applying acupuncture. My first patient was a woman in her early 40s with right shoulder pain. Two years before she injured it in an accident. In spite of many medications and physical therapy she continued to have moderate to severe pain most of the time. After examining her it was clear there was no major nerve damage or complicated tissue abnormality. I suggested we try acupuncture, something she had never done before. Because of her sensitive nature and cautious concern I used only two needles. She sat in treatment for ten minutes and it was over. Two days later I saw her and she reported no pain since having the treatment. Several days later, at the end of the two-week session, she was still without pain and, of course, delighted.

After providing acupuncture for hundreds of patients over the years I am convinced of its value. It is rare to see a quick excellent response to one treatment. Nonetheless most respond well to a series of treatments. In conjunction with stretching and strengthening exercises it is often very useful. Although I do not use it for many other conditions I have patients who have reported to me its value. The medical literature is becoming much more supportive in the use of acupuncture for many medical conditions. Eventually this will be a treatment modality that is taught to not only physicians but also nurses, initially for pain relief, but eventually for much more.

Acupuncture is very safe. There have been reports of adverse effects. Local infections occur rarely. Hepatitis and other infections have been reported to be spread by acupuncture. Now the needles are used only once, they are sterile and very safe. These are solid bore needles with only a point, not a shearing knife-like effect present with injection needles, and therefore much less likely to damage tissue. At times bruising can occur as small and, rarely, large vessels are punctured. There are reports of lung collapse and pneumothorax, but these are quite rare. Compared to injection side effects the incidence of complications is very low.

Homeopathic Treatments

Homeopathy is the creation of Samual Hahnemann in 1796. He was a pharmacist before attending two medical schools. Concerned about the harm done by conventional practice at the time, be began to explore dilute herbs, minerals and animal extracts.

A primary principle of Homeopathy is "Like cure like," referred to as the Law of Similars. What is found in nature that causes a set of symptoms may also reverse such symptoms when present in a patient. This is the basis of vaccination as well, though with miniscule amounts of the offending organism.

Hahnemann and several close associates experimented on themselves and their patients. Over the years several textbooks have been written that document how to prescribe a remedy. Homeopathic training requires astute observation of appearance, speech, posture, mood, mind and response to examination. The primary emphasis is questioning a wide range of symptoms, times of day occurrences, effects of food, and general mental patterns of behavior. Many symptom complexes and conditions have been identified by its practitioners to respond to homeopathic remedies.

The remedies are diluted and percussed (shaken), a process called potentiation. Often the dilution process goes beyond the point where identifiable molecules of the original substance are present. This defies the usual scientific understanding of the value of Homeopathic remedies, a major reason for rejection. However recent studies suggest that there is a memory of the original substance that registers with the diluting substance, usually water.

Scientific studies have produced mixed results. Some recent research has been compelling, but many studies have not supported the benefits claimed. Conventional medicine considers homeopathy no better than placebo. There are many practitioners with stories of healing after conventional medicine was shown to have nothing more to offer or had resulted in severe adverse effects. Homeopathy should be considered for any chronic disease and some acute disease because it is safe, inexpensive and potentially helpful.

There are few adverse effects. I have occasionally heard stories of temporary distress requiring bed rest and food restriction for up to a few days. Usually there are no adverse effects. The most common complaint by conventional medicine is that it may delay more effective treatment. I agree that professional diagnosis and a clear discussion of potential problems are necessary. Once a condition has been defined and reasonable discussions have occurred Homeopathy should be pursued in those who are interested. It is especially worth considering in those who are very sensitive to medications, herbs or foods. Anyone with chronic disease should consider homeopathy, whether responding to other treatments or not.

The Role of Spirit In Health And Disease

The greatest contribution of Integrative Medicine to the practice of modern medicine is its inclusion of spirituality. The emphasis is broad, not specific. Practitioners are encouraged to explore and discuss basic principles of spirituality, not a specific religion. There is not a coercive effort to be spiritual but encouragement to pursue it if so inclined. In most of the major meetings on Integrative Medicine organizers provide discussions and training in effective prayer, mindfulness, and meditation.

Integrative medicine seeks to override medical and societal disinterest and rejection of spirituality. Our healing elders were very spiritual, however modern medicine has only recently begun to respect the role of it. In the last 100 years medicine has more completely embraced the definition of science as observer and mediator of the physical plane, excluding the psychological and spiritual domains. As it elevated the status of the objective scientist it denounced the value of what it could not measure. Scientists assumed that if you could not measure the role of the emotion, mind and spirit, it did not play a role. In general this has been a major advance also forcing science of the heart and mind to be developed more convincingly.

Fortunately methods of measurement are being developed to study spiritual influence on healing disease and establishing well-being. The medical field is finding a new respect for religion and spirituality that will lead to a more intelligent and effective use of them.

The other main reason for excluding spirituality has been societal. There is resistance to religion dictating direction by faith and dogmatism. Political differences have risen about the role of religion in society. Many people assume that religion and spirituality are the same. Fortunately there is a trend to separate these. Integrative medicine is, at least in part, at the forefront to do so. Some medical practitioners are now being encouraged to support patient's practice of religion and spirituality to enhance healing.

Spirituality is the study of the forces that feed and guide our lives. It encompasses the energies of sources of life, higher motivation and meaning. As we consider the value of life from the perspective of the soul we begin to identify fruits of the spirit such as kindness, caring, compassion, goodwill and generosity. We know these are part and parcel of the substance of healing as well as the intelligent mind and mature heart. As we respond to the needs of those who are ill we can invoke the energies of these forces.

There are many ways to invoke forces of spirit into the healing process. I suggest the cultivation of three qualities of the inner life: loving kindness, loving understanding and loving dedication. These are real energies that heal us from deep within. They help us cooperate with the source of our life, however we best understand that to be.

Loving kindness is the recognition that we have the capacity to be gentle with ourselves and those around us. Life is hard in many ways. We want to be able to control its harshness with our own strength of muscle and might. These efforts help but fall short of the complexities of thought and feeling, attachment and desire. Kindness recognizes the need to respect the life within ourselves and others. Each of us hopes for similar goals of health and wholeness and needs to be willing to do our part to accomplish them. Kindness elicits cooperation and a willingness to work together, to be more tolerant of differences and more willing to quickly forgive ourselves and those with whom we interact.

Loving understanding involves the role of the mind. It engages our capacity to consider the many facets of important decisions and close relationships. We usually do not know the reasons why others treat us the way they do, especially negatively. As we learn to explore the impact of prior experiences, especially fears and frustrations, we begin to connect the dots and threads of events that led to statements and actions that affect us. Loving understanding is our effort to allow more time to learn about ourselves and others before making conclusions or taking actions we may regret. We do not need total consensus to act but may find it worthwhile to include a larger part of the whole, and look for the larger good that is growing through us. Loving the truth and following its direction leads us to greater understanding and healing.

Loving dedication is the force that helps us define noble endeavor. We need to want to be well for good reasons, not just to avoid discomfort, dysfunction and distress. Too often the goal of healing is to return to what we thought was better health before the disease or accident occurred. However, overcoming disease to resume the same habits of self-centeredness and neglect, at least in some ways, is of little value. The life within wants us to be useful in some way to those around us. We need to want to be well for a reason that serves a greater purpose that supports or benefits more than ourselves. Loving dedication helps us to identify the strengths, skills and talents we have developed that can serve the needs of others. Sometimes we are called to mainly serve family and friends. However many of us are called to reach further, to the groups to which we belong and those whose path we cross. All of these opportunities, lovingly embraced, invoke a healing presence and power. Healing may not occur until we are part of an effort to extend and express ourselves to those around us. Healing does occur as we identify with and express the best within us and within those with whom we live and serve.

How To Assemble A Healing Team

Each of us needs a physician. We need regular exams, laboratory tests, x-rays and other tests especially as we age. We need to have someone available when we are ill and worried about the problem. Many of us do fine with only a physician for medical care. A growing number of us need specialists, adjunct health practitioners and counselors. Especially when serious disease occurs we often need a team of healers.

Finding the right physician is usually by word of mouth. We ask our family and friends whom to see. We listen, ask questions and maybe schedule an appointment. We should at least ensure the presence of credentials, that the individual is licensed to perform the tasks we need. For minor problems this is less of an urgent concern. For serious, chronic or debilitating problems more checking should be done. Fortunately most physicians can be Googled and basic information easily obtained. Asking the professionals we know will often give us valuable feedback and suggestions for how to find the information we need.

The sign of a competent physician is the presence of intelligent, caring behavior. The usual forms should be filled out and questions should be asked. An exam should be performed. An initial appointment may not allow for a complete exam but if not done recently should be offered soon. The first task of a physician is to diagnose the problem or at least offer possibilities of explaining the symptoms of concern. There should be time for questions. Physicians have their own time schedules and some include more time than others. The style of care should be satisfactory or else keep looking. Complex conditions require a thorough discussion of current concerns and clear suggestions for what to do about them. A cheerful demeanor, an eagerness to serve, a willingness to listen carefully and respond thoughtfully are basic qualities to expect.

Reasonable expectations of professional care are necessary as with most of our life and relationships. I know one physician who says at the outset to give him one year to see what he can do to best influence your health. Most people decide long before that if they will continue care or go elsewhere. Access to the physician or support staff needs to be available especially for urgent questions or changes in health. After-hour access needs to be available as well or at least knowledge of the process of receiving help needed. I always inform a new patient that I do not provide hospital care but that a hospitalist will be on call for such care if required. Most receptionists have basic information about the care provided and how to obtain it under different circumstances.

When problems are serious we need a team. A comprehensive team includes a primary care provider, appropriate specialists and possibly many other special care providers. Often the basic medical team includes chiropractic care, physical therapy and personal trainers. Some people have a chiropractor as primary care provider, many of whom can provide basic medical care or at least know when to refer for physician care. Which ones are chosen depends on prior experience, personal preferences and the nature of the problem. Depending on the interest of the individual it is also worth having available an herbalist, acupuncturist and/or a massage therapist.

The more serious the problem the more likely I will also suggest consulting a counselor, a pastor or rabbi. At times I recommend a healer and even an intuitive counselor. These practitioners may enhance healing in remarkable ways and often make a difference. There are many ways to learn about the nature of our medical problems and conditions. The more receptive we are to the range of possible agents of healing the more likely we will find what we need.

The ultimate healer is within ourselves. Many of our problems are physical in nature and can be treated effectively with physical means. However serious problems require outside advice and expertise. Most of all we need to learn how to mobilize our inner knowledge of who we are, why the problem is occurring and what we can do to heal ourselves. No one knows ourselves better than we do. The inner healer may need the help of experts to accelerate healing with medication, surgery or other treatment. The wisest course is to ask for help, take what is appropriate and apply the steps that can be done. The task of personal assessment, insight and healing can be pursued concurrently if necessary. The ultimate answers often unfold slowly as we sincerely state the need to know. In serious situations we always need patience, persistence and a deep dedication to love ourselves and those around us.

For greatest effect, we need to be in charge of our own care and captain of the team. It is important to ask for what we need and how to accelerate the healing process. We are the ones who make the final decisions and should accept the responsibility for doing so. Self-honesty and integrity are great allies in helping us connect the dots and see the sequence of events that led us to where we are. Courage to confront our blind spots helps expose weaknesses and unresolved issues. Compassion heals what is missing or misapplied. We are never alone with the presence of love, wisdom and joy that is the source of our being. As we awaken to the presence of these within us we mobilize healing power.

Mobilize the Will to Heal

Chapter 19

How to Pray for Healing and Wholeness

Prayer is seeking aid from spirit, however we best understand that to be. Its origin is a deep yearning to commune with our source of life and use it to better our lives. Prayer is primarily considered a practice of religion and is an element of all the world's major religions. I suspect it predates organized religion and was a part of the larger life around us and within us from the beginning. Any sincere appeal for help must come from deep within us if we expect it to make a difference. What we call prayer is not as important as recognizing that it is a useful exercise of heart and mind for help and healing.

There are many benefits of prayer and many studies to verify its use. Studies report the value of prayer in hypertension, heart disease, survival rates, endocrine and immune function, substance abuse, cancer, eye operations, operation recovery, pain, anxiety and depression.

One of the most publicized studies involved people admitted to the hospital coronary care unit with a heart attack. Admitted patients were separated into two groups, one prayed for and the other not. The groups were randomly chosen and studied for almost one year. The patients, the staff, the doctors and the investigators did not know who was in which group. In the prayed for group 85% had a good course in the hospital as compared to 73%

in the non prayed for group; 14% of the prayed for group had a bad course as compared to 22% in the control group. The recovery rate, complication rate and length of hospital stay were all reduced in the prayed for groups.

One of the most powerful studies with prayer was done on individuals with HIV. Gail Ironson is a psychologist and psychiatrist at the University of Miami. She conducted research on 100 patients with HIV. Predictors of improvement were based on HIV virus count and CD4+ T-cell levels (helper cells) over a four-year period. Those who did not believe that God loved them had markedly worsened CD4+ T-cells at a three times faster rate than those who believed that God loved them. Those not prayed for had three deaths in the group of 20, and those prayed for had no deaths during the time of the study.

Although there is a distinct trend away from churchgoing, recent research indicates great value in attending rather than not attending church services. Studies show that 91-98% of the public believes in God. Eighty-five per cent pray, 73% feel close to God, and 72% approach life on the basis of religion. Well over a thousand studies have been done in the past decade. Strawbridge and colleagues studied over 5,000 adults over 28 years. They found that attending church regularly decreased the risk of dying by 36%. Caucasians who attended church weekly lived an average of seven years longer, African-Americans about 14 years. The risk of dying during the eight-year follow-up was 50% higher in those who never attended compared to those who attended more than once per week. A biochemical connection is positive with interleukin-6 levels, an immune system secretion associated with greater stress and dysfunction.

I was raised in a Christian home and attended a private religious school for several years. I attended church frequently and participated in the services in various ways. However I do not recall learning how to pray, when to pray or how to know that prayer is working. These are basic questions that are worth knowing for those interested in pursuing the use of prayer. I have continued to be interested in prayer and have attended seminars about it over the years. There is much to learn about the nature and use of prayer for the spiritually minded and interested in mobilizing the power of healing.

The distinguished American psychic, Edgar Cayce, had a great deal to say about prayer. Essentially, he said that prayer is talking to God and that meditation is listening to God. These are both simplistic summary statements and yet they embody the attitude that many assume about prayer and meditation. Edgar himself demonstrated a reverent attitude for prayer, recommended it often and used it frequently himself. Records of his spiritual suggestions to others provide a rich reservoir of life changes and healings in body, heart and mind. Mr. Cayce made a frequent admonition that we seek to be a channel of blessings to others, and that itself will lead us to greater health and well-being.

When I first began to search for guidelines to prayer I attended a conference about it at the Edgar Cayce Foundation in Virginia Beach. I learned about the many types of prayer including prayers of forgiveness, healing and gratitude. At the end of the week I had a dream in which I was in a huge New York City ticker tape parade. I was sitting in a convertible on top of the rear seats, as is commonly done by officials in parades. As the car turned a corner, the words boomed out, "Hooray, he has learned how to pray!" Yes, the joke was on me! My higher self was saying this has value but don't overdo it. Prayer is helpful, but we are not celebrating a major success, simply a way to lead a better life that many have chosen over our long history.

Shortly after my medical training I had the great opportunity to meet and study with Olga Worrall. She discussed and demonstrated laying-on of hands healing. She and her late husband, Ambrose, were studied by several researchers including those at UCLA and John's Hopkins. Many of their healings are well documented and inspiring. In their writings they describe prayer in a succinct discussion of how and why it works.

Ambrose states that prayer is analogous to how we think, and that thinking sets in motion subtle energies that determine whether we call forth healing energy or disease energy. We have the capacity to choose the ways to higher living such as honesty, integrity and serving others. Or we can choose to be anxious, irritated, rebellious and resentful, which will lead to further distress, disappointment and disease. These choices are always available although they may not seem to be by those stuck on feeling distressed and depressed.

From Dr. Robert Leichtman and Carl Japikse we learn that prayer is a natural part of the spiritual minded person. It is one of several skills of spiritual practice and can be used often for guidance, insight and healing. The steps for effective prayer start with a quiet devotion to the source of life within, the soul. We call forth our conscious awareness of its presence in our life, and our gratitude for the many ways it watches over and aids us. We accept its love and dedication for us. We invite its presence to help us cleanse and purify ourselves of fears, doubts and worries. We state our allegiance to its plan and agenda for us and re-dedicate ourselves to its purposes.

With prayer we can focus clearly on our current needs, the efforts we have made to meet them and the need for further help at this time. With continual applied effort we become familiar with the subtle ways of life unfolding within and around us and the healing energy associated with them. With gratitude for its presence we develop a deepening relationship with the spirit of healing. This is how prayer can work for us.

Types Of Prayer Available To Us

There are prayers for intercession, healing, forgiveness, gratitude and joyfulness. Most prayers are used to get us out of trouble, for someone or something to intercede in our suffering. We usually do not ask for help until we need it. We do not ask for help when we begin to slide away from commitments or react with irritation, impatience and stubbornness. We wait until mired in the mud of fatigue, disease and despair. We often indulge our likes and dislikes but not higher meaning or the consequences of our decisions. Prayers of intercession may be helpful, but asking for help before we need it may be even more effective. Asking for help at the beginning of the day, the beginning of certain relationships and the beginning of certain projects is the best time to pray.

Healing prayers are very common. Prayer often leads to healing when it is accompanied by honest self-assessment and re-dedication to our better selves. Most of the time healing prayers do not work as fast or as completely as requested. However such prayers may well re-awaken us how to take better care of ourselves, how to repair mistakes and confront unresolved differences. Prayers for healing are more likely to work when associated with the sincere effort to do the right thing. Unfortunately there is a strong urge to pray for what we want, what feels good and what will relieve us of any discomfort or suffering. God is not Santa Claus and spirit has its own agenda of priorities.

Effective prayer is when we pray for what is possible from the perspective of spirit. Prayer is more likely to work when we ask for what is reasonable to be energized and made manifest, rather than the fears and worries we have about our problems. What we attend to attracts energy. If we focus on frustration we attract faltering and fatigue. If we complain and blame we energize the inner critic and its tendency to harass and harangue. If we resent and seek revenge we stir up self-recrimination.

The more we define the healthy focus the more likely we create the wholesome good that is needed. We need to be well for a reason, to fill the obligations we've chosen, confront the challenges we face and develop the relationships we're in.

Prayers for healing require forgiveness for harm we have done and help for what we failed to give. The ancient prayer of the Our Father says that forgiveness begins with ourselves. Unless we apply the need for review and revision to ourselves it will be hard to do so to others. As we sincerely revise how we could think, feel and act better we attract insight on how to do so. As we admit where we have been wrong in what we did or didn't do, the more we call forth greater kindness and gentleness toward ourselves.

As we forgive ourselves we are more likely to see the real need to forgive others. Our feelings and thoughts are connected to a vast history of events since the time of birth. Patterns of reacting, judging and expressing who we are have healthy and unhealthy aspects to them. Forgiveness is a crucial lever of lightness than keeps us balanced on the teeter-totter of life, active and moving toward our mature self. Forgiveness is how we learn to love ourselves in spite of what is missing and undeveloped.

Prayers for gratitude seem less often used though not because they are less important. The value of gratitude is to reinvigorate our sense of hope and confidence we are moving in the right direction in our relationship with higher self. Gratitude helps us rise above disappointments, discouragements and a diminished sense of self. If we are too hard on ourselves we belittle our capacity to perform and relate well with others and the work that lies before us. Just as we need meal breaks to reenergize the body, we need gratitude for the good we feel, see and do to boost our mood and mind. Life is meant to be celebrated. Our good deeds need to be recognized and rewarded, to be increased and expanded.

No one knows the real efforts we make as much as ourselves. So we cannot rely on others to recognize the difficulties we overcome to do our best. Of course we also know our own falterings and failings. These need attention but not rejection and condemnation as much as correction and rededication. Of course overdoing self-recognition can lead to self-centeredness and self-absorption. Genuine gratitude can help us stay on track especially when extended to higher parts of self. The source of our being will keep this awareness balanced if we allow it do so.

Gratitude leads to joyfulness. As we are grateful we see the greater expression of the delights around us. The kindness of strangers, the enjoyment of flowers and the resilience of nature become more apparent as we notice them. Beyond attending to the good we feel and see we can add the energy of thankfulness to the source from which they come. Prayers of joy connect us to the choir of contributors of the music and art that we enjoy. These energies in turn empower us to surge into the challenges and turmoil of the day with renewed purpose and power. Gratefulness generates awareness of the goodness and greatness of life.

How Do You Know If Prayer Is Working?

It is hard to prove the effect of prayer, but the possibilities are intriguing to ponder and very real to those who experience them. A personal experience is the most convincing. While working at Meadowlark I recall one individual who was having a most difficult time. He was not physically ill but had accumulated frustrations in his family and work relationships. At the Retreat Center he did not relate well to the other guests. He was emotionally isolated and disappointed with himself. One morning during my meditation time I prayed for his well-being and sought to see how I could especially help him that day. At the session that morning the group process proceeded as usual. However right after the class he approached me and said, "I know you love me." He was reassured and appreciative. I affirmed his comment but thought about whether this had been set in motion by my own efforts to attend to him in prayer. I was not aware of anything I said or did with him during that session in particular. Something special reached him that was beyond me.

At times the only way of knowing the effectiveness of prayer is the inner strength of purpose it instills. One of the most inspiring dream about prayer occurred to me a few years ago. I dreamed that I was at an ideal healing center quite like Meadowlark. There was a lightness and brightness about the center, its activities and the staff working there. Everyone seemed fully dedicated and delighted with the work they were doing. At one point they gathered in a circle when I heard the leader say, "We have room for one more." I joined hands with them and he proceeded to say "May the light from the center of all that is good shine to us and through us." To which I usually add, "And to all those I meet this day." I use this prayer often to re-center myself at various times during the day. To me, it was a burst of boldness that brings brightness with every use of it.

Effective prayer can especially be enhanced with attunement to the soul, our center of well-being. A daily routine of prayer increases the power of it. Like the practice of piano, art or a favorite hobby, the more we do it the better we get. The simplest method may be to call forth a healthy memory of the person involved, knowing that what has been can be again, and more. For some it may be best to commune with the ideal pattern of mind, heart and body, and then energize it with our own spirit. For others it may work to invoke the "Center of healing known by God." There are fountains of healing that have been created by the many over the millennia of time. Those before us have created reservoirs of healing that a sincere devotion with a genuine need can reach at any time. Let us believe it is so and trust its presence to work its way through us.

The bottom line of benefit is the results we obtain. By their fruits you will know them. Studies have been done and will continue to measure the effects of prayer. On a personal basis we need to verify if prayer works for us. As we apply it to our questions and challenges we should see positive results or learn new ways to use it.

Why Doesn't Prayer Work More Often?

Prayer does not work for those who are filled with fear, anguish or despair. These are hard to overcome with a quick change of heart unless there is an unusual connection to the center of our being. Long habits of worry, anger or resentment darken the memory of how to ask for help. Strong memories of dismay and distrust dampen and, over time, destroy the best of intentions. These must be addressed before prayer requests can be expected to be realized.

Prayer does not work for those who do not do their share of the work required. Spirit adds to the effort we make. A teacher or a tutor will be less than willing to help a student who does not show signs of effort and study to understand the assignment. Unless you are a Tom Sawyer, friends are not interested in helping you paint the fence let alone pay for doing it. When we do our part others are willing to pitch in. And spirit works the same way. Like a loving parent and friend it is always available to add to the efforts we make.

Prayer does not work when we become distraught or overwhelmed by tragedy. Personal problems are at times unexpectedly traumatic. In a state of shock it is difficult to contact our higher self. Initially we must stop the bleeding heart and mind. Trauma forces us to consider how to make sense out of what we just experienced. We must understand circumstances before we can open our hearts and minds to solutions or prayerful requests for aid. There must be a shifting of gears to rise above the situation to consciously be receptive to inner help. This can be done and many learn how. The more skilled we become the more quickly we can move to a higher part of ourselves, even in an emergency.

Excess sympathy for the suffering of others can also obstruct our effort to help with prayer. When already filled with our own problems and obligations we can easily reach a limit. Overload occurs at times because we are too sensitive to the suffering of others. Sympathy is actually an instinct of identifying with the suffering of another. It can be helpful but requires energy to express. Sympathy is often taking in the feelings of distress whereas compassion is expressing love to heal it. Compassion is the use of the higher heart and mind to be of help in constructive ways. Prayer can connect us to the source of compassion to express it more fully when needed for others and self.

Prayers for large problems in society often do not respond readily. In our age of 24-hour news networks we are more aware than ever of serious problems affecting large groups of people. The suffering is easy to see and feel. The instinct to react and respond is deep within us. If over attended, concern for huge issues will drain us quickly and worsen our own health. As we invite more suffering than we can handle we easily become overwhelmed. In this state we add to the problem instead of the solution. As individuals we need to focus first on the problems in our own immediate world. These are the ones for which we are most responsible. As we grow in skills of spirit we may be led to larger fields and groups of endeavor and responsibility.

Certain prayers are designed for large groups. Using such prayers can at least give us the sense that we are doing something positive instead of complaining and blaming or being afraid and frightened. Humanity has a long history of crises, turmoil and tragedy. From these problems have arisen great prayers of inspiration and support to address them. These prayers include the 23rd Psalm, The Our Father and The Great Invocation. First to self, then to those around us. The practical focus for prayers of large groups and events is for those in positions of authority and decision. We can pray they do the greatest good for the greatest number. Not for self but those in need and the principles for which they stand. The greater the attunement the more likely our efforts will reach the larger groups to which we belong and those who lead them. In these ways we can mobilize the power to help heal the groups to which we belong, small and large.

The Great Invocation is especially designed for current global problems. Its can add positive energy to the world and also protect us from the fear and despair of major human suffering. This is The Great Invocation as written by Alice Bailey:

"From the point of Light within the Mind of God, let light stream forth into the minds of humankind. Let Light descend on the earth.
"From the point of Love within the Heart of God, let love stream forth into the hearts of humankind. May the Coming One return to earth.
"From the center where the Will of God is known, let purpose guide the little wills of humankind, the purpose which the Masters know and serve.
"From the center which we call the race of humankind, let the Plan of Love and Light work out, and may it seal the place where evil dwells. Let Light and Love and Power restore the plan on earth."

Guidelines For Effective Prayer

Effective prayer starts with a need to express ourselves more fully. There may be a need to heal, a need to help someone we care for deeply or a need to celebrate the good we have received. The real need is usually more than our own suffering or that of another. The missing energy is often a strength that is missing such as courage, confidence, self-acceptance, love, wisdom or resilience. When we pray for a specific quality of life or energy of expression we attract memories and energies of having done so or examples of others. Remembering what has worked before helps mobilize the higher energy we need now. Imagining the help from a mentor, counselor, hero or heroine can also impact the effort.

These steps can be used to make prayer more effective:

1. Identify the need: healing, forgiving, resolving a problem, appreciating or creating a new effort.
2. Choose a strength most likely to fill the need: enthusiasm to start the day with positive expectations, compassion for self or another, courage to confront a person or situation, insight to know what to say,

love to enrich a relationship, or wisdom to know how best to address current concerns.

3. Commune with the higher self to learn its perspective of the current issue: what is its priority, its understanding of the causes involved and how best to cooperate with it.
4. Dwell on the ideal condition unfolding with the strength chosen and present in all those involved including self.
5. Repeat this sequence regularly, one to three times per day for one to four weeks; you may choose how many times per day and for how long.
6. Look for signs of improvement, the evidence of things unseen and yet possibly connected to your efforts
7. Be grateful for all that is received and all that is good whether noticed or unnoticed, obvious or subtle.

Chapter 20

Linking the Heart and Mind to the Soul

Meditation is an excellent way to explore and develop the spiritual yearning for the higher self. Along with prayer, the study of sacred scripture and responsible living, meditation is one of several tools that help us tread the spiritual path. The primary purposes of meditation are to enhance our direct experience with the source of our lives and to integrate it with our daily challenges.

Meditation slowly became a Western practice in the 1960s. The seeds were planted several years earlier by a few extraordinary teachers from India like Paramahansa Yogananda. The West has had its own enlightened teachers of prayer and meditation including Alice Bailey, Joseph Leadbeater, Charles Filmore and Earnest Holmes. Meditation has come to be a universally accepted method that transcends religion and yet may be promoted by it. In the West, most religions are far more likely to encourage prayer than meditation, with which there are similarities and differences.

Meditation is primarily a practice of self-reflection, inspiration and guidance from within. Like prayer, meditation begins with the recognition that there is a source with which we can commune. Meditation is more of an appeal to the higher mind than the heart. It is a means whereby we learn how to love with the mind, the higher mind that can commune with the source of beauty, harmony and comprehension. In meditation we access greater understanding about the issues we face. Rather than mainly relying on friends, family and experts for how to handle conflicts, meditation encourages the use of our inner resources of insight, intelligence and understanding.

Within each of us is an immense reservoir of past experience. We have a basic set of skills gained and lessons learned. As we dwell on the higher memories and energies we call forth the capacity to be creative in our hopes and expectations for how to improve our life and those with whom we live. More than the memories available to us there is an inner yearning for inspiration and illumination. The inner yearning helps us activate the urge to learn and grow. As we strengthen this connection we mobilize the meanings and purposes of our life. As we expand this relationship we energize the personality with a larger perspective and the ability to bring it into the priorities of the day.

Many studies have shown the values of the practice of meditation. Stress, pain, blood pressure, respiratory conditions and even cancer have been shown to improve with consistent uses of meditation. Anxiety, panic disorder, depression and post-traumatic stress disorder respond as well. The physical and psychological benefits are possible with relatively little training but regular practice. To relieve such problems is reason enough to pursue meditation. More compelling reasons to practice meditation include the desire to reach beyond ourselves, to help others with their problems and contribute creatively to the relationships and work we have to do.

There are many ways to develop the skill of meditation from the simple to the more comprehensive. Some would have us mainly become relaxed and choose a single focus, such as a candle, the breath, a word or a mantra. Others require strict guidelines for posture, attentive breathing and chanting. These have value for those who are overwhelmed by excessive worry, fear, anger and frustration. However excessive attention to the body is more likely to be boring and ineffective for those sincerely seeking a more creative expression of living.

I have experimented with many types of meditation from the East and the West. The most effective method I have found is taught by Robert Leichtman and Carl Japikse. It is an active form of meditation in which the mind is encouraged to participate in the process, that it is a vital piece of the whole, not to be shut down or left behind. The mind and heart are necessary to serve as a platform on which renovation and innovation can land for effective expression. There is a process of stages that help us detach from our usual concerns and commune with our higher nature. We deliberately detach from the body, emotions and mind and yet keep them active for integration and application of the inspiration drawn forth.

Stages of Meditation

Relaxation, detachment, attunement and application are four stages of active meditation. Meditation is like any major endeavor. There are steps to take to pursue it well. Just like taking advantage of an appointment with an exceptional expert on a particular issue, we need to prepare ourselves to decide what to do with wisdom of the connection made during meditation. We need to consider the best use of time available. Will the wise one know all our concerns and just show up or do we ponder our questions? If the time is limited what do we most need to ask? What are the higher priorities? How can we be most alert during the time set aside? What attitudes of expectation, respect and carefulness are most appropriate? During the meeting do we remain silent and only listen or do we present ourselves with genuine needs to address? After we hear a response to our questions do we just leave or express appreciation or pursue the questions further? After a thorough discussion how do we best show gratitude? After leaving the wise one do we just enjoy the feeling of the experience as long as it lasts or do we consider ways to implement what is learned?

Relaxing the body is the first stage. We relax to put the body at ease and diminish its concerns so they do not distract us. Of course this means setting aside the time needed, finding a quiet place, a comfortable posture and a brief relaxing ritual. It is helpful to choose the same time and place on a daily basis. The body does accommodate to routine and will actually anticipate a meditative period by automatically beginning to relax on its own. That is why a period of time should be set aside, initially anywhere from 10-20 minutes, though this varies from person to person.

A relaxing routine is helpful, especially when beginning. It can be as simple as recalling a favorite site in nature or the memory of awakening in the middle of the night, nicely relaxed and somewhat refreshed. A breathing exercise can be helpful, such as saying the words "I am" on breathing in, and "Relaxed" on breathing out. Making too much of the relaxation phase detracts from the main goal of meditation, which is to increase our conscious awareness of our whole self, not just the physical body. Eventually, this phase should be relatively easy, almost automatic and brief.

Detachment is the second stage. It is the process of not only letting go of current concerns but also rising above them toward our true identity. The purpose of detachment is to move beyond our usual worries, frustrations and plans of the day so they don't interfere.

Detaching from the body is one thing, detaching from the heart and mind is another. It can take more time because we invest so much of our energy in how we feel and think. To do so it is helpful to review our recent common expressions of distress, worry and concern. It is worthwhile stating that we are aware of the feelings we have and acknowledge their presence. But we also need to be aware that we are more than these as we seek to reach higher than the body of feeling. We appreciate the value of our feelings and honor their presence but recognize that our heart is connected to the heart of God. At this time we seek to dwell in the presence of it. We rise above the personal concerns so that we make room for the higher, subtler sense of a quiet loving presence.

At times detaching is very difficult when we are consumed by strong feelings of worry, guilt, sadness or anger. The tendency is to replay recent events, words spoken, what we saw, heard and felt. As these feelings and memories are played over and over we empower them to dominate our attention. To move beyond them may require a major effort. At some point we must confront ourselves with practical steps that can be taken and be satisfied with that while we seek to reach our inner being. We must be determined to find greater strength of new resolve within. We must move from one room of attention to another room of creative possibilities. We turn off the light in the room of fear and frustration and turn on the light in the room of new hope, new healing and new learning. We appreciate the presence of the goodwill of the heart and consciously decide to move beyond it.

As we rise above the body of feeling we enter the body of mind. This is the body of thinking, analyzing, problem solving, planning and preparing. It is filled with many events and relationships, successes and failures, incomplete understandings and certain gained awareness. The mind has the capacity to be aware of itself as an observer and learner of life. More than just noting the details of the events through which we pass, the mind also is the main actor in our roles of life. We are a parent, child, worker, friend, relative and more. We detach from the mind when we reach for our higher identity. We call forth the fact that we are a child of God, of Life and of Love. This is our real self, our whole self, our true identity. We appreciate the value of the mind, choose to rise above it and attune to the indwelling spirit as best we see that to be.

The third stage is attunement to the higher self. The source of our life has many terms including love, spirit, or soul. We become comfortable with terms used from our childhood, parents, religion, friends and peak points of learning. The term we use is not as important as the recognition that there is a source with which we seek to commune, that it is innately our friend, who is wise and loving. This indwelling friend is our vital ally in solving turmoil, overcoming challenges and opening new opportunities for creative expression.

A sincere appeal opens the doorway to the treasures that are present. A sense of devotion and dedication cleanses us from lower drives and helps us be attentive to higher ones. Gratitude for help to be received draws us inside the room. Reverence for the source opens our higher self to the mind, heart and body to receive what is given.

It can help to have a specific need. Stating a need provides a focus of attention around which ideas and solutions may gather. At times, the best invocation to spirit is to request an increase in a talent, skill or strength needed. This may include a request for how to be more forgiving, tolerant, compassionate, reverent or joyful. At other times, we may be filled with a compelling urge to act, to take a stand with ourselves or another, to walk through fear, expand a relationship or start a new project. All of these can be pursued with active meditation.

The goal in meditation is to discover the higher priorities and seek to fulfill them. Many are taught to surrender to whatever the higher self may send us. At times this is helpful, especially if overwhelmed with an intensely stressful set of circumstances. However it may also be far too passive. The higher intelligence seems to work best through us when there is a particular need to know and skills through which it can speak. There is an agenda of the higher self and it needs a mind, heart and hands through which to work. The more skills present the more ways it can be expressed.

Upon reaching the higher self we commune with it for a period of time. This may be brief or longer depending on the need and time available. Often it is best to accept the connection made, dwell with it and then begin to return or put it to use in some way.

The fourth stage is application, the conscious awareness of how to use what is received. With a renewed sense of approaching the day with reassurance and a greater sense of inner guidance, we can project calm, creative energies to be more available. Most of us know the main events and people with whom we will interact. It can be of value to rehearse the day, at least briefly, with greater patience, kindness, resilience and more ready reliance on the support available within. The Quakers call it meditating with our feet, following through with aspirations to acts of goodwill. Applying what we gain in our quiet time grounds insight and energy into useful activity. Until we integrate what we have gained we do not engage the subtle energy awakened. The cycle is aspiration, ascension and application.

How do we know that our efforts are worthwhile or even moving in the right direction? My experience in practicing, teaching and listening to my patients who meditate is that miraculous changes are very rare. Most improvements are slow and subtle but also very apparent over time. *By the fruits you shall know them* we are told. So it is worth looking for the signs of greater degrees of calmness in the face of turmoil, quicker capacity for forgiveness when unfairly criticized and more access to common sense for important decisions. At times the best sign of progress is a growing sense of contentment in spite of difficult relationships, incomplete projects and deep disappointments. We become more aware of doing our best and proud of it. We look forward to tomorrow to start again to add life, cheerfulness and goodwill wherever we can.

A Healing Experience With Meditation

One of my patients related this experience to me:

"I lay on the basement floor, my face against the cold cement, hoping to alleviate the anxiety that was eating away at my body and mind. I wanted to somehow find relief, even if it was for a few moments. It seemed as if I had tried everything, from herbal remedies to prescription pills, but nothing had worked. The once healthy and successful man I was seemed to be rapidly deteriorated before my own eyes.

"'Have a great day, Mr. Energy,' the doormen would say as I rushed out of my apartment in the city each morning to get to work. After forty years of building and maintaining a dental practice in Long Island, I was still operating at full speed. Even moving to California was not enough to slow me down. Rather than retiring or relocating my office, as most people would have done, I chose to continue running the practice. This was not an easy task—red eye flights back and forth across the country every other week, leaving my wife and children for appointments, and constantly running on overdrive—which would have its consequences. Although my hard work and commitment led to many opportunities from radio interviews to being the founder of the Holistic Association of New York, it was only a matter of time before my body would start to show warning signs of exhaustion.

"To the rest of the world I was perceived as someone who was almost superhuman, a man who had the perfect balance of obtaining his career goals and an ideal family life. But secretly I knew I was slowly falling apart. At the age of sixty-nine, I was still holding tightly onto my practice. It was everything I had ever wanted and the result of unwavering dedication throughout the years. But this routine now consisted of going to my office in New York nine days out of the month, intermittently, while trying to maintain a personal life in California. Countless hours were spent sitting on airplanes and waiting in airports. Somewhere along the way, going to work became a chore, causing me to go beyond even my physical limitations.

"The result of all this was catastrophic but unavoidable. I could no longer sleep at night. Although my body was burned out, my mind would not let me rest. Even when I was at home I seemed to have lost interest in my usual hobbies. After adhering to a strict diet for over forty years, in this time of desperation, I pushed aside all my values. I started drinking alcohol and taking prescription drugs, but even that did not assuage my anxiety. The worst side effect, however, was not being able to smile or laugh. I no longer felt any pleasure in the life I was living. My once lighthearted soul was taken over by dread and worry. After almost four years of enduring the arduous schedule I realized it was time to let go.

"On March 13, 2008, I sold the practice. I then decided to go back to my daily routine, which included yoga and meditation to heal naturally without any drugs or medications. I began to go to the Vedanta Temple in Montecito and immediately felt right at home. The temple peacefully sits atop a mountain, directly overlooking the ocean. The inside consists of beautiful woodcarvings, and although I was the only person there, I felt the spiritual vibrations of others who meditate and pray there. As I meditated, the sunlight shone through the windows bringing me a sense of warmth and serenity. For the first time in almost a year I smiled in celebration of life."

The Limits of Meditation

In gardening it is necessary to dig the holes for seeds to just the right depth. If you go too deep the seeds won't reach the surface. They will remain dormant until life is possible above the ground. If the seeds are too close to the surface they will dry up too easily and not unfold. If left on the surface they will burn up from the sun or be eaten by birds or other hungry insects. So, too, with meditation there are healthy and unhealthy ways to approach it.

Going too deep into meditation for too long a time may disconnect us from the life we are living. There are times to retreat from life, to look deeply for a new view or to reassess priorities for the purpose of reaching higher.

However the rhythm of life often pulls us back to the current issues and obligations. We do not learn patience by avoiding conflict or peacemaking by withdrawing from a relationship before its time. We do not learn forgiveness by shutting down all chances to work through the differences with family or work relationships. We do not learn tolerance or cooperation with others by disconnecting all communication. At times any of these may be temporarily necessary, but only to allow breathing space for a chance to return, re-connect and re-commit. At times we grow beyond our relationship with key individuals and groups but only when the work is finished, not before.

Even the spirit minded can be misled. There are many levels of self-deception. Meditation can be one of them. I have seen more than a few students who pursue meditation so earnestly they create further trouble. A few become physically ill with back pain, sleep and fatigue trouble. At one time I had a husband-wife team as patients. Both of them had physical disabilities of the use of their hands preventing them from practicing their career. They were both students of a teacher from the East who himself was disabled. His legs were unusable from excessive meditation, from sitting prolonged periods of time, cutting off the circulation and eventually paralyzing them. This is not the spirit of meditation.

At times I've seen patients who have been confused, disoriented or agitated from meditation. Usually they were trying it out too vigorously and too seriously. Some students of meditation approach it with an intensity that is disruptive to their body. To start any endeavor with enthusiasm is admirable. Sometimes there is a tendency among some students and teachers to over-emphasize one or more aspects of meditation that may limit its values to us. There are some whose primary purpose is to raise the kundalini, a Hindu word referring to the subtle energy of the body. To obsess on any one aspect of meditation is usually not healthy.

Meditation can help guide us through the turmoil and challenges of relationships. Relationships never end. They can be made worse. We can turn them into fiery pits of hell. And we can put them on a shelf, for a lifetime or more. Yet the pull of life will always be toward completion, a deep regard for the inner life and unique contribution of each. Meditation can help us fulfill our commitments to each of those in our life and the larger causes that they serve.

The Ultimate Goal

The ultimate goal of meditation is to bring heaven to earth. The goal is not go to heaven and stay there. Many consider the goal to be to detach from life and its problems and not have to return, to live in bliss or peace and not having to be part of the problems on earth. I think we should see meditation as a tool with which to draw upon the highest elements within us so we can improve the life we live.

When first learning anything there is a need to focus. There is often a tendency to overdo. Like the old teeter-totter, our inner nature will continue to take us back and forth, up and down, until we find the balance that works best. When done in healthy ways, meditation will connect us to the inner being that will help us move from the end that is high to the other that is low until we find the fulcrum. Eventually we learn to see the source of the balancing point and can re-connect to it whenever needed.

There are many steps and several levels to the wise use of meditation. Like with great music, we are meant to soar with the high notes of lovely harmonies and then bring them back to the lower ones, mixing and lifting. We are called to experience the heights of beauty, peace, calmness and serenity, and then bring them down to the work of the day, mixing and swirling until it, too, is an expression of delight, enjoyment and fulfillment. In these ways meditation can mobilize the power to meaning, healing and wholeness.

Chapter 21

The Healing Effects of Movies, Music and Art

The fine arts are sources of healing because they inspire our creative impulses to translate beauty, harmony and joy into real life circumstances. The fine arts include a wide range of artistic expression from acting to painting to poetry and writing with many versions of each. They often bring the higher perspectives of life into usable expressions of color, music and drama. They provide means by which we can see greater depths and heights than our usual five senses. They help us explore hidden recesses of the nurturing heart and fertile landscapes of the curious mind. The fine arts expose the mud and slime of things as well as the promise and potential of enlightened genius awaiting the awakening kiss of the creative fires.

The fine arts have been an avenue of inspiration, reflection, insight and healing for eons of time. The Greeks used theater to tell the great stories of heroism and tragedy. They knew the need to tell the stories of the struggles of heroes and heroines from hardship and obscurity to strength and success. Hercules was born strong in many ways but still had to demonstrate how to use his skills of living wisely because physical strength was not enough. He had to awaken his strengths of heart and ingenuity of mind to match the foes he faced. The twelve labors of Hercules continue to be a source of inspiration to the aspiring agent of healing 3000 years later. Today we need to learn how to confront immense problems that also seem insurmountable to us. We each need to find ways to adjust, adapt, and start again, over and over and over, as we climb the ladder of growth, learning and worthwhile being.

The genius of Shakespeare and those with him expanded the public forum of theater as an enlightened way to expose the foibles of society and the many sad, silly ways we handle them. The Shakespeare team explored the turmoil of leaders, their many deceits, revenge, fears, doubts and courage, as examples for how to respond to the tragedies of our own lives. His comedies continue to show us how to laugh at ourselves with the complicated convoluted circumstances we create, and the marvelous synchronizing results that can still occur with reassessment, sincerity and humility.

One of my early experiences with theater was attending a performance of "The Gates of Rashomon." This is a story about the assault of a noble woman on her way to Kyoto, the revered sacred site of healing in Japan. The Rashomon Gate is a prominent entrance to Kyoto just outside of which a noble woman is attacked by a fellow traveler. At the trial, four people testify, the victim, the accused, a witness aid to the victim and an individual with psychic ability. Each has a compelling story but the observer is left to decide the truth of the accusation without a jury or proclamation from a judge. We are left with having to decide ourselves what happened for the purpose of awakening our own heart and mind.

Life is similar. There are many points of view. We are obligated to learn as many as possible and decide the best actions to take. Disease is an attack on the body. However causes of disease arise from multiple factors, each of which needs exploring. Often a single cause is not identified. Whatever the cause of disease and healing, it must be pursued like justice, making the best of what we know without knowing it all.

The cause of our problems is never as important as what we do about them! The cause of mud on the floor is not as important as the need to clean it up. The cause of debris on our dishes or dirt on our clothes is not as important as the need for us to clean them. The cause of fear, doubt or anger in ourselves is not as important as the willingness to heal them. Fortunately no matter the cause of a disease, there are many sources of healing upon which to draw. Great art provides an innovative way to heal ourselves and the life in which we live.

Movies are the modern means of the masses to experience the theater of our time and the healing experiences that come through them. Few movies deal with disease directly; however many of them deal with insight, healing and transformation.

***Cocoon* is an excellent example of how to re-awaken hope when the forces of aging seem to have taken over.** The story is about a few older folks living in a retirement community. They are dealing with aging bodies, long relationships, extended family problems as well as the diseases of dementia, heart failure and cancer. Of course, they also represent old ways of dealing with new problems, ways of childhood or early life that do not apply now. A few of them stumble onto a swimming pool of a neighbor. The more they play in the pool the healthier they become, and it awakens a genuine excitement in living. It turns out that the regenerating energy is radiating from large seed pods in the bottom of the pool. Eventually they discover them to be fetuses from another planet inadvertently left behind but soon to be retrieved. In the end the retirees are offered the chance to fly with the aliens to the planet of pod origin. They can continue to be young and healthy or choose to stay behind and let nature run its course of progressive disease and death.

Cocoon is a marvelous metaphor of the real energies that can be life saving in body, mind and spirit. It helps us think beyond the usual to the extraordinary and yet possible. We age in many ways besides the body. Too many of us age by adding to our fear and doubt by becoming worried and weary instead of confronting the problems with courage. We add to our guilt by belittling ourselves daily instead of accepting the forgiveness available and the lessons learned. We add to our depression by developing sarcasm and cynicism instead of finding reasons for hope and optimism. Each of these has a second and third generation of dysfunction that lead to progressive darkness, identifying ourselves as incomplete, incapable and unredeemable. The relationships in Cocoon exposes these patterns and provides ways to rise above them. Some of the characters succumb to their fears, others stay with their families out of sympathy for them and a good number take the leap of transformation.

***Cocoon* inspires the yearning to find and follow the answers to aging in body and mind.** It reaches beyond the fantasy fountain of youth by suggesting that there is a place that we can go to claim new life. Spaceship travel to another planet is fantasy. The implication is that we travel in consciousness to another part of ourselves and the world within to which we are connected. Those who are willing are invited to take the trip. The requirement is the choice to leave behind the current habits of activity, mood and mindset. That does not mean that we disclaim our past or who we are. It means that we reach above them to find further aspects of ourselves. It starts with believing that something special is there. It opens our imagination to explore the sky within us. It requires releasing ourselves from the attachments we have so that we find a better focus for our purpose and meaning.

The obvious suggestion in inspired theater is to reach within and above to higher realms of thought and action. As we are shown how it can be done we are encouraged to invoke the source of the majestic muse within ourselves for the issues at hand. Whether raising a family, working to support a family or pursuing a personal mission, there is a vision toward which we can aspire. As we reach one we are led to another.

Many movies are of magnificent value. Any art that draws upon genuine sources of inspiration have universal appeal for lengthy periods of time. Some of the older ones continue to be sources of moving inspiration and creative healing. These include *The Wizard of Oz, Gone With the Wind, Casablanca, Fantasia, Amadeus, Star Wars, Raider of the Lost Ark* and *Harry Potter.*

The story of the hero and heroine is the story of the spiritual person, each of us, seeking to follow the spiritual path. It starts with an obscure individual, yearning for a better way, impetuous, impatient and immature with current circumstances. With seemingly few options available and simple steps ahead, like the yellow brick road, life then becomes cloudy, murky and intimidating. The passage of time is accelerated to show consequences of right orientation and aspiration.

When lessons are learned doors open, when lessons are not learned suffering occurs. Obnoxious, angry tyrants are frighteningly powerful but only up to a point. Fear, weakness and withdrawal do not advance progress. Courage, cooperation and persistence win the day. Many steps are taken and eventually success is gained. We find home, friendly folks and the usual chores ahead with hope and hardiness abounding around us. Life is calm again for a while. This is our destiny though often experienced with many pitfalls, delays and detours.

Using good movies for healing often means identifying with a favored character and behaving as if you are that person. Such an exercise does connect us to the part within that has similar seeds of strength waiting to be explored and expressed. The main characters connect us to the hero within or expose the truth we need to see. A genuine interest in learning generates healing energy especially as we integrate the new model and apply it in the life before us.

Music Magnifies Healing

Music is a field of life that draws forth many healing energies. It is a kaleidoscope of enjoyment, delight, calming quietness, courage, confrontation, thunderous exclamation and healing. Music can ennoble us to higher hopes and nourishment or distract us to experiences that stimulate our urges of pleasure and excitement. Music is more than in the ear of the beholder. Studies have been done on plant life that show it, too, has a very sensitive nature alert to its environment and its caretaker. Plants grow toward certain kinds of music and away from other kinds. Classical music is like pixie dust fertilizer, brightening everything in hearing range. Brash music is like a harsh wind, destructive in its tantrums.

The beauty of music is real and objective, not just personal whim and preference in the ear of the beholder. It is worth exploring and studying what kinds of music promote health and healing and what kinds disturb and distress us. Such insight can help us heal faster and prevent distress from leading to disease as well as increase our joy of living. One of the most intimate experiences with another is listening to wonderful music together.

I first became aware of music applications several years ago. Suggestive Accelerated Learning Training (SALT) is a program that was studied and applied at the University of Iowa to train language teachers how to use music to enhance learning. Studies were done at elementary and secondary schools. The researchers found that those who were exposed to baroque music between language lessons learned the language 2-3 times faster than those who were not exposed to the music during the learning sessions. Sandwiched learning with music made a difference to most of the children without prior music training.

While working at Meadowlark Retreat Center I began to experiment with music and healing. I conducted several classes using music as means of renewal and regeneration. The class started with a focusing exercise of writing a list of current issues, challenges or relationships to improve. A single item was chosen for the purpose of the session. We meditated briefly, requesting guidance from higher self. A piece of music was played during which participants were encouraged to listen with the issue at hand or use the imagination to invite a person in question to listen, too. After the music ended each participant was encouraged to write down whatever occurred during the music time for reflection and insight.

One of the most interesting experiences occurred to a woman who sought healing with her sister. She had not spoken to her sister in over seven years. This particular evening we listened to Mozart's "Eine Kleine Nachtmusik." At the suggestion to invite someone to share the music she invited her sister to listen with her. During the music she felt that they were together at night, in the winter, window-shopping for Christmas presents. They had a wonderful time together like the good times they used to share. After the event, writing and reflecting, she said that it is time to contact her again. The inspiration of Mozart helped to re-awaken the core of concern, the real bond in the relationship with her sister. She was receptive to it and chose to act on it.

Another patient reported a dream one morning involving the healing of a legal matter. In the dream he was in a courtroom setting. He heard a statement made from the plaintiff, thought of how to counter the contention and advised his lawyer how to push it. Suddenly, the music of an old song came to him: "Who cares if the sky cares to fall in the sea. Who cares what banks fail in Yonkers. Long as you've got a kiss that conquers..." It was the song that he and his wife enjoyed when they were courting. It changed the whole sense of himself with the current issue. He realized that the fight in court was for his lawyer to handle, that the situation would work its way out. He had a better focus for himself and his creativity than to be consumed by this legal matter. The old favorite song connected him to the part of himself that enjoyed life. The music helped him heal the frustration and worry that was distracting him from the writing work that was his career and love of life.

I remember a time when a music piece became part of a healing event for me. There was tension about how to integrate a new staff consultant at Meadowlark. She was a psychic intuitive who was being promoted strongly by the administrator of the center. The board of trustees was invited to hear her speak and then asked their comments about her capacity to help guests in the program. Most of the board was not impressed to a major degree. The administrator was very disappointed but not about to be overridden. She decided to essentially replace the board instead of changing her view of the individual. I suggested caution but was worried that her involvement was not an addition to the program and might actually harm it. Guests were being encouraged to write the psychic for guidance instead of writing to their own higher self, our usual approach and the most healthy one.

My routine at the time was to nap after lunch for a few minutes. One noontime I awoke from the nap with an old song on my lips, "The More You Get Together." It goes like this: "The more you get together, together, together, the more you get together the happier you'll be. For your friends are my friends and my friends are your friends. The more you get together the happier you'll be." And it was true that we had many friends together, especially the staff of the center. I made some efforts to meet and chat with her but was reluctant to do so vigorously.

Receiving guidance is one thing, following it is another. At one point a close friend of mine, an emergency room physician who used to hold my position there, confronted her with her limited view of me. She interpreted his comments as a breach of trust from which we did not recover. If I had followed the guidance I had received, we may have been able to repair the relationship. It was a downturn in the direction of the clinic which did die within a few years later. Was the music more than a warning or also a source of healing?

A few years ago I became involved in a difficult legal matter. I was accused of not diagnosing prostate cancer soon enough. The chart notes did not support a thorough assessment of the situation although the patient had been informed that he had an abnormal PSA blood test. I could see that this would be a long, difficult experience to go through. I consulted the insurance company that was very reassuring in providing all the support needed. I consulted my mentor/counselor. He predicted a settlement, that it would take time but would work out to my benefit in the long run.

Within a few nights I had a dream, during which I was taken to a large room in which were a large number of books. I went to the back row of one section and out dropped a piece of music. It was a piece written by a singing nuns group and had been one of my favorite pieces. During my college years I began to play the autoharp. It is a small, handheld harp of 36 strings that easily fits in the lap. I played it to renew myself during the heavy study times of medical school and residency. My favorite tunes at the time were a collection of pieces written by this group of singing nuns.

The particular song I re-discovered is entitled "It's a Long Road to Freedom." This is the refrain, the main part I remembered: "It's a long, long road to freedom, a winding steep and high. But when you walk with love and the wind on your wing, and cover the earth with the songs you sing, the miles fly by."

It is a very optimistic song and was very reassuring to me. It requires the choice of being loving, kind, caring, compassionate and cheerful, to self and others, day by day, in spite of the worries and concerns. It became a song for me years ago. I took it deep into my soul, and at a time of need it came forth, a well-timed flower in my garden of spirit. It lifted my mood more than anything else at the time. Whenever I would worry about the problem I would review the words, re-dedicate myself to what is most important and feel deeply the support available. Music can transcend turmoil, reach into the core of our being, above the clouds into the light of healing and wholeness.

Music reaches parts of ourselves that may be hard to access with our usual efforts. It is a different route than the common conscious focus from which to understand, analyze and plan courses of action. The type of music in our repertoire of experience makes a difference. Whether calming, strengthening, forgiving or peacemaking, healing music is available now more than ever before. No matter how difficult the time the choice can be made to find music to add to all of our other efforts. Music renews and regenerates the power of healing.

There Is An Artist In Each Of Us

I have very little art ability. From an early age my imagination did not work when it was time for art class. Finger painting was fun but did not produce anything worthwhile. I learned how to paint by the numbers and even enjoyed it, though obviously barely creative. Nonetheless, a new spark was triggered when I first went to work at the Meadowlark Retreat Center.

For the first time I was near outstanding art museums with first-rate masterpieces a short distance away. A dream helped propel me toward the art nearby. A favorite staff member at Meadowlark pulled me aside one day and said she had a dream for me. The dream occurred by the beach. She was standing on the sand when my father appeared playing a violin. When finished playing he told her that I was to include more art in my life. She was quite confident the dream was actually a nighttime experience, not a typical personal dream, but a visit of my father to her to encourage me toward the world of art. I took the suggestion seriously and began to visit the museums and concert halls in the Los Angeles area. Each visit was uplifting and exhilarating. A whole new world opened up to me.

During this time an opportunity arose to travel to Greece with a close friend, an emergency room physician. We visited Epidaurus, the site of the famous healing centers started by Aesculapius about 1000 BC; they lasted 1500 years, well into the Roman times. That is quite a run!

In visiting the center we heard, read and reviewed the stories of many healings, of the lame walking and of the dying being healed. The entrance over this healing center was *"Pure must be he who enters here."* Someone later added, *"To be pure means to be clean of heart and mind."* This is a great way to approach any new effort to learn and grow: To ask for new light and love and life; to cleanse whatever holds us back in terms of distress, doubt and despair that clog and distort the better nature of ourselves.

A suggestion was often given to a guest seeking healing to sit at the foot of a statue of a certain god and learn from his or her strengths. They had quite a selection at the time, a wide variety of forces of nature, personified as human strengths, though with their weaknesses as well. There was Athena, the goddess of nature, like the alert deer, swift, vital, cunning, resourceful, watchful; strengths that can heal the weak, tired and foggy-brained as well as plan deceptions. There was Poseidon, the ruler of the seas, often depicted as the charioteer drawn by several powerful horses, representing the power of strong feeling and vigorous passion, as well as uncontrolled rage and unhealthy obsession. There was Apollo, the god of love and healing, often seen with a lyre for music. He represented the healing energies of compassion, insight and contemplation, especially for the overly distressed and guilty.

When I returned from the trip I remember approaching the main office at Meadowlark. On the counter of the office desk was a stack of art books from the great museums of the great artists of the Renaissance, the Impressionists and others. They were about to be taken to a garage sale. I was immediately intrigued and asked for the price. The outrageous cost was a dollar a piece. So I plunked down a $20 bill and took the stack. Within a few weeks I had gone through most of them and put a course together using the books as focal points for healing, like I had learned at Epidaurus. I realized that a great painting is like sitting at the feet of a hero or heroine of life, that we could learn about ourselves, heal ourselves and be re-inspired from deep within. Great art is connected to the source of life, a fountain of vibrant energy and a wellspring of new ways of living, thinking and feeling.

During some of the early classes I conducted there were two incidents that were particularly striking. They both led to outstanding examples of insight and healing that can occur in just one session. A middle-aged man chose a painting by Rembrandt called *"The Polish Rider."* The rider was a military officer in a colorful uniform, alert and engaging. He got involved in the painting with the suggestions given, wrote down his conversation with the Rider and then shared it with us.

He said that initially he was looking for how to be more masculine, confident, stronger in his career and key relationships. However he was surprised at the discussion with the Rider. It turns out that the Rider discussed with him the value of being considerate, sensitive and kind, and that these are actually more strengthening than the usual expressions of control, firmness and forcefulness. That a real man also is able to be aware of his sensitive side and express it when needed. He said these comments helped him accept the feminine part of himself that he was having trouble integrating into his personality. It was a quite revealing and inspiring experience for him.

The second one involved a woman in her early forties. The issue of concern to her was how to respond to the inner urge to be a mother. She was without children of her own, living with a man who had two older children from a previous marriage and he did not want more.

She chose a painting of a nicely dressed woman, looking over her two young daughters at an outdoor picnic on a lovely grass lawn near a large old tree. During the visualization exercise she was asked to enter into one of the individuals in the picture. She found herself choosing one of the children. The resulting dialogue between the mother and child engendered a delight in being mothered. She felt deeply reassured about herself by the presence of this loving mother energy.

When she came out of the visualization exercise she said she was surprised whom she chose to enter. She thought she would enter the mother to experience the love for her children. Instead she entered a daughter. She decided that it was not mothering she needed to experience as much as mothering herself more, that as a child she did not get enough attention and support. Along with counseling sessions she felt this helped her resolve the need to have a child. She realized she needed to be a better mother to herself and that this would lead her to fulfilling creative activity.

Some psychologists specialize in using art for counseling. At Meadowlark we had one woman on staff specializing in art counseling. She conducted group sessions where direction was given to draw or paint for expression. With guidance she helped many explore themselves in revealing and healing ways. I recall one woman in the class who expressed her current problem in the form of a devil-like figure, with horns and red colors, though not mean and angry. When asked to paint her ideal self, her higher self, she drew an angel-like figure with lighter shades and a happy expression. When asked to bring these two together to further a relationship between these disparate parts of herself she drew a pleasant looking woman, a human figure, with colors from each of the other pictures. Though few experiences are quite so dramatic many found insight flowing forth with the effort to give form and color to the inner life. For some this is an excellent way to evoke healing energy to coordinate and collaborate the higher and lower parts of ourselves. Color on paper by the non artist can be a way to mobilize the healing we need to see and express.

Writing Is Healing For Many

In these days and times we all learn how to write though few of us become writers and only a tiny number choose it as a career. Nonetheless, many more of us can benefit by writing about ourselves. The inclination to write a diary begins in many childhood and teen years. The digital age has increased this capacity for many of us to do so. I confess that this was never a strong impulse with me, although, I did attend a writing dialogue workshop many years ago that was a wonderful experience.

***The Intensive Journal Workshop* is a book that provides guidelines for how to have an inner dialogue with yourself.** It was written by Ira Progoff, an American Jungian psychotherapist. Based on this approach he developed a weekend workshop that took participants through a step-by-step process of self-exploration. There is little talking and little sharing even at the end of an exercise. Most of the time is spent writing initiated by a brief visualization exercise to awaken the creative imagination. The weekend is structured to begin slowly with simple explanations and exercises. One lesson is to address turning points in life. This session was followed by questions to consider how certain roads not taken may still be available. The last exercise was a dialogue with wisdom and the most compelling one for me.

I followed the suggestions to relax and proceed down a well to an underground stream. Suddenly, "I am at a train station about to board, saying good-bye to my current companion of the time. I go on a quick journey that leads to the church in which I was raised. I find myself in the front pew. Not many others are there. It becomes clear that the ceremony is not going to happen until I approve of it.

"In the pew with me are several mitres, the elaborate headdress of a bishop. [This church was the bishop's church, where he celebrated mass on the major holy days]. Unless I am willing to allow him to have his hat the ceremony will not proceed. I chose to do so. The procession of the bishop and his retinue proceeds down the aisle. When the tabernacle [which contains the Eucharist host, the bread for communion with the Christ] reaches me, I am entranced by it and the experience ends."

The main meaning of the experience was to confirm my newfound authority to spirit from within. I had the authority over my life that a bishop has over his congregation of several priests and thousands of parishioners. I was elated with the humor of the situation, which is usually a hallmark of genuine insight for me. It did turn out that the relationship with my companion ended soon after that.

Writing is a way to externalize what is happening within and around us. The writing creates a mirror in which we can see ourselves more clearly and decide what to change. The mirror of our feelings, reactions, fears, doubts, hopes and plans are there for us if we but look and see. Most of us keep looking at the same patterns of thought and feeling, the same rooms, the same contents and in the same way. Instead we need to explore the other rooms in the mansion of who we are and what is in them in new ways. A well-designed writing workshop can do this, and we can do this on our own if properly motivated to do so.

Studies show that writing can help facilitate healing in a wide variety of disease. The diseases that research has shown to benefit from writing are AIDs, breast cancer, asthma and rheumatoid arthritis. Even the common cold occurrence decreased in college students who followed a study designed around writing. A writing expert I know personally researched the benefits of writing to aid those with depression and other somatic illnesses and found it to be healing.

I have used writing in many workshops with a variety of topics. Often I will recommend brief writing exercises that initially request listing current issues, then choosing one for the session we are doing. A specific focus of concern mobilizes attention and healing energy. The energy is always available but it often requires a cup to catch it, a mouth to pour into it and a stomach to digest it. One bite at a time is more likely to bring noticeable effects than attacking a huge problem head on, which may be like trying to eat a whole chicken.

Lawrence Spann is a Physician Assistant and Ph.D. in Literature. He conducts writing classes to learn about, express and confront ourselves. He provides a few guidelines the main one of which is to "Write, write, write, to your heart's content." He often gives a starting seed thought, a favorite quote or provocative statement about which to focus. Mostly he creates an atmosphere of eagerness to explore yourself and make a connection to the wellspring of exuding life. The smallest event, sound or object is a story waiting to be written. His writing workshops are invigorating and delightfully enjoyable. This is the enthusiasm to approach our inner artist yearning to be felt, seen and heard. For further interest read the book *Blood on the Page*, edited by Chip Spann and Jan Haag.

Writing is an excellent way to record dreams. Dreams are unfolding every night but few of us develop the memory capacity to recall and record them. One of the best ways to remember a dream is to have a pen and paper at the bedside. It serves as an act of faith that something will be remembered. The writing externalizes the otherwise ephemeral energies of thought and feeling being processed throughout the evening.

Writing is an excellent way to set goals. Goal setting is a superb way to set forth the ideal direction in which we seek to grow and learn. There are several steps that can be taken for such a project. The first is to write out briefly the ideal state of body, heart and mind, the ideal use of the five senses, major feelings of emotion and skills of the mind. Then write the ideal state of key relationships and key issues of current concern. By considering the ideal state we commune with the soul and its agenda for us.

After we describe the ideal state we move to practical steps that can be taken where we are now. The more these are written out the more likely we will implement them during the day. The more we write the more likely we act and the more likely we will integrate the ideal into the real. If this is a persistent consistent expression it can lead to further unfoldment in every aspect of living.

Poets also see the real life around us, at times with an extraordinary perspective. Some of them see the seeds of life in the worst of the dark and suffering and even in the ugly, the angry, and the hateful. Life is like the poem by Ralph Waldo Emerson entitled *Music*:

Let me go wherever I will, I hear a sky-born music still:
It sounds from all things old. It sounds from all things young,
From all that's fair, from all that's foul, It peals out a cheerful song.

It is not only in the rose. It is not only in the bird.
Not only where the rainbow glows. Nor in the song of a woman heard,
But in the darkest, meanest things. There always, always something sings.

'Tis not in the high stars alone. Nor in the cup of budding flower,
Nor in the red-breast's mellow tone. Nor in the bow that smiles in showers.
But in the mud and scum of things. There always, always, something sings.

The Art of Living

Each of the arts of acting, music and dance is an avenue of many healing energies. They convey a wide range of experiences that express lower and higher aspects of ourselves. The two masks of theater are the sad and the happy faces. Life is full of tragic distress and discomfort, depression and despair. But it is also full of comedy, kindness, cheerfulness, cunning and delight. It is worthwhile for everyone to find at least one aspect of the arts to draw upon regularly. For some it is more effective than counseling, prayer or meditation for receiving guidance and direction. The arts have a way of bypassing our conscious mind and preconceived ideas about life to allow greater renewal and regeneration. We each must find our own unique and creative way to participate in the great drama of life to a fuller extent. We are designed to learn and master the art of living. Inspired music, masterful movies and enlightened art are means whereby we can mobilize the power to do so.

Art is filled with stories of life with many ways to enjoy and learn from it. It is also a distinct avenue for learning the art of living. The pursuit of the art of living is similar to the artist seeking to explore and express the exquisite beauty of love, wisdom and joy in paint, dance and theater. In psychology these are referred to as signature strengths, in religion as the fruits of spirit and in life as the joys of living.

We can learn from all of art from the simplest to the most complex. It depends what you are looking for, why you are looking and what is in front of you. Going to an art museum or reading an art book or going on line to find art can be easy, fun and enjoyable. However if you want to use art for learning, healing or inspiration, it helps to focus on an issue through which the beauty can shine. It is like going to your doctor, counselor, minister or rabbi. It helps to develop questions about the issues, consider the options available and listen carefully to the advice given. With art we bring the harmony, perspective and inspired energy to the issue at hand and look for creative ways it stirs us. Great art can lift us through if we prepare ourselves to be lifted.

The art of living and healing is finding the quality, attribute or energy that is most needed. The list is long. I suggest that the main categories are love, wisdom, strength and joy. Each of these has other categories, any one of which may be a main category for you. For instance, love is often expressed as kindness, calmness, caring and compassion. Wisdom is seen as intelligence, reasoning, remembering, understanding and creating. Strength is present in confidence, courage, determination and persistence as well as restraint, patience and purpose. Joy is often felt as delight, gratefulness, friendship, and any celebration of living. And these are just putting the toe in the water of the art of living.

Great art is inspired from the deep well of inner truth that has universal connections to the source of life itself to which we are all connected. As we seek to find our indwelling source of self we can use the outer signposts that others are shining toward us as a way to proceed. Great art can be such a trigger when approached with a need to know and genuine appeal for guidance. Entering into the art we view can awaken the art of life slowly unfolding within us. A masterpiece self-portrait is being painted as we go about our life with the many choices we make and the responses we express to those around us. As we eagerly embrace the events of the day we become an agent of the art of living and mobilize the power of healing for ourselves and those around us.

Chapter 22

Finding Nature's Healing Energies

Nature is the presence of life within which we live and move and have our being. Nature's abundance is immense and dynamic. Nature is the source of all our food, air and water. These are the basic ingredients of survival. We don't live without them. Fortunately we have learned how to produce abundant supplies with the raw materials of nature, soil, seeds, and water. Making them available for all is a major goal of humanity. The specialty of integrative medicine is helping us bring forth much more research and use of the healing effects of nature's abundant supply of vitamins, minerals, herbs and hormones in our food chain.

I was surprised to find out that about 70% of all the medications in use today are from nature or nature-inspired. The rain forests are filled with many unexplored healing agents and the oceans are just beginning to be examined. Our future is bright beyond belief in our relationship with the abundance of nature!

The most widely used medications today are the statins. Some enlightened individuals decided to study Chinese medicine. They learned about red yeast rice, a red yeast that grows on rice. It has been used for thousands of years to treat people with heart disease. Researchers identified the active ingredient, tested it, found that it decreases cholesterol and, more importantly, lowers inflammation levels in the body (inflammation causes the red blood cells to become sticky and thus clot more easily increasing the risk for heart attacks and strokes). Statins are the most prominent medications in the cardiovascular field at this time for treating and preventing heart disease. It has side effects in part because of suppressing co-enzyme Q10 levels, occasionally liver strain and cognitive dysfunction. There are no known problems from the yeast itself.

The healing capacity of this planet's nature is still in its early phases of development. There are many ways that nature already helps us heal the heart and mind with the plant kingdom. Besides the physical uses for healing there are subtle uses of these as well. Samuel Hahnemann founded **Homeopathy** 250 years ago by studying and developing the subtle energies of plants and minerals. He showed that these not only help heal physical ailments but also emotional and mental ones. Edward Bach created the flower essence treatments, commonly called **Bach remedies.** He discovered the healing effects of flowers for a wide range of mood disorders from anxiety to depression to loss of control and emergencies. Homeopathic and Bach remedies have been used by thousand of practitioners over the years. Beyond the physical uses of these remedies are many more ways that nature nurtures our heart, mind and spirit.

What Do I See In A Tree?

One of the most compelling teachers during my undergraduate years was a rabbi. I signed up for his class, Introduction to Mysticism. We read about William James and other great agents of transformation. We discussed religious experiences from around the world. Near the end of the semester he offered a 24-hour intensive sensitivity class. Because of the limited number allowed and a large number wanting to participate he drew names out of a hat to decide who would be involved. My friend's name was chosen first and mine was second. It was the first time that I participated in intimate sharing of deep concerns and yearnings. After the session my friend and I visited the Rabbi's family and learned about Yasodhara Ashram in British Columbia. It was their retreat center for renewing themselves.

Based on the traditional learning centers in India the ashram was founded and run by Swami Rhada. She was a dancer in Germany before WWII. Her family helped several Jewish families escape the camps during the war years. Though they were harassed, frightened, questioned and stripped of clothes during the abusive interviews they continued to help where they could. After the war they emigrated to Canada. While working as a clerical secretary one day she walked by a bookstore. In the window was the face she recognized from a recent dream. He was the author of a book and a teacher from India. She purchased the book, wrote the author and was accepted as a student. She lived on his Ashram in northern India for six months. Due to her having already learned many life lessons she finished her training in a short period of time. She took vows of poverty and service and became an expert Yoga teacher. Soon thereafter she returned to Vancouver and began to teach what she had learned.

Swami Radha developed a class called The Straight Walk. It is designed to learn basic principles about healing, direction and the spiritual perspective of life. It is an eight-day class limited to 15 or so participants. There are three sections to it. The first was simply a walk outside in nature for twenty minutes. We observed what we saw, wrote it down and then re-gathered. Swami Rhada led the group discussion then focused on one participant at a time asking questions about the list of observed objects. Whatever was listed as seen in the walk was pursued as a point of discussion until some kind of meaning was found.

When it was my turn I asked a direct question, "Should I finish medical school or strike out on my own and do what I most want to do, become a spiritual counselor." She said, "You're almost done. Finish school, complete what you've started, then you can do what you want." I bypassed the list that was meant to expose the questions life was asking of us. I knew my question and she gave me a direct wise answer that has served me well.

When I went back to the list my first object seen on the walk was a tree. It became apparent that the tree is more than a tree. It not only has leaves, branches, a trunk and roots, it stands for my appearance, what sustains me, the core strengths and roots of nurturing life within me. The Straight Walk helped me understand more about the events, relationships and opportunities that arise in my life. The outer events are the surface of deeper larger issues, the meaning of which can be found with asking questions, searching for answers and exploring the depth of current issues. I learned that we are each meant to be explorers in the realms in which we live. We are armed with various tools sufficient for some tasks and challenges, insufficient for many others.

The purpose of the walk of life is to develop and refine the tools we have to express the love, wisdom and joy that resides and radiates from within. Every object, event and relationship has a meaning to us based on who we are and how we see that life around us. Each one is an opportunity to express the best within us. Our inner nature is a powerful force of insight, inspiration and illumination waiting only for us to find it and use it for those we serve. The Straight Walk is a means to awaken the inner higher nature for mobilizing the power of healing. It is a vast abundant resource of insight and guidance.

Communing With Nature's Spirit

From the Straight Walk experience I developed a class for healing and self-awareness. I first taught the class at Meadowlark Retreat Center and thereafter the adult education program in Santa Barbara. We began with a brief meditation during which we asked for guidance from the higher self on what we need to know about a current issue. The instruction was to walk outside the room around the grounds. I suggested that each pariticipant look for a site to sit and ponder something in nature, take up to 20 minutes pondering its significance and then return to the room. The instruction was to write what happened, what was seen, heard and felt. Then we gathered in a circle, shared our experiences and discussed it further. We helped each other look for connections to greater meanings, broader perspectives and steps to take.

One of the most compelling events occurred to a middle-aged man. He chose to sit in front of an orange tree that had a grafted branch of a grapefruit tree. During his pondering time he came to see how the tree accepted the grafted branch and freely shared its nurturing energy as with all its other branches. He felt the spirit of nature as a life-giving force that embraced life in every form.

While considering these impressions he reviewed his relationships with his current wife and her two children. From the beginning of his relationship with his second family he recalled the children's efforts to engage him further, to deepen their relationship with him. He become more acutely aware of how he declined their entreaties to become part of their lives feeling he was not responsible because he was not their father. During this brief session he came to realize that his attitude was not in line with the spirit of nature that embraces the life it is given. With remorse and re-dedication he chose to realign himself and begin to be a father to these children who wanted and needed him. He was relieved to identify his new mission and uplifted all of us with his insights. Nature exposed his own deep urge to love the ones in front of him and he chose to do so.

The stories of nature are abundant, real and ready for use, awaiting only the enquiring heart and mind to mobilize them. Nature is not only a source of dynamic physical energy, cycles of change and constant regeneration, it is also filled with resources to awaken us to the spirit of life.

A St. Francis Moment

Many years ago I read *The Secret Life of Plants* by Peter Tomkins. It described the ability of plants to express themselves in many ways. They grow toward music they seem to enjoy and away from music they do not, like loud rock music. They are also affected by the life of their owners, so that they exhibit withdrawal when there is distress in the life of the owner and increased exuberant energy when the owner is having a good time and enjoying living.

More recent research shows that the roots of corn saplings emit a clicking sound. When they are exposed to a similar sound they grow towards it, attracted to one of its own kind. On the other hand some plants secrete chemicals that slow the growth of other plants. Science is slowly documenting the intricate ways plants communicate with each other and those who listen.

Nature is filled with healing energy from the animal kingdom and the spirit within them. Since childhood I have been friends with many family pets. We had birds, cats, dogs, hamsters and chameleons. The most unusual was the chameleon. It was given free range in the five-foot planter between the dining and living rooms. As a child it was intriguing to see its color changes from yellow to red to green to brown depending which color of plant it was near.

The closest pet to me as a child was Trix. He was mixed breed dog of unrecognizable origin that followed my older brother home from an alley one day. He left at night but always returned for food and eventually became a much-loved loyal pooch. Most interesting to us was that he learned how to hunt pheasants and ducks quickly. He retrieved many birds over the years to more than pay his way. My older brother and I would argue over her got to hold him in the duck blind when it was very cold, and he was a constant companion of the kids in our family for many years.

Over the years my own family has had four dogs, the last two German Shepherds. They have been the best guard dogs and very loyal to family. Although intelligent and disciplined they have been sensitive and supportive whenever there were difficulties or distress in the family. The last one with us, Micah, is especially a healing influence whenever needed.

Fortunately there is growing use of dogs to serve society. Certainly the police use them for potentially difficult individuals as well as searching for missing children and pets. They serve the blind but also others with various disabilities and needs. Their use as companions rivals that of friends and family. It is not uncommon to see a patient suffering from major grief over the loss of a canine companion.

One of my most cherished memories of communing with nature occurred on a sunny afternoon in the lush hillsides of Wisconsin. One day while working on the horse ranch of the Pain Clinic I took a stroll in the woods. I was reading a wonderful book about the broader nature of life and became somewhat tired. I lay down under a lovely large oak tree and dozed off for several minutes. When I awoke there were several animals all around me -- horses, cows, goats, and birds. They were all within touching distance. It was like we were all the best of friends. The horses were eating the grass and looking toward me as I awoke. The birds were very close, chirping away. The goats were a little further off but only a few feet. It was quite exhilarating. I suspect it occurred in response to my willingness to learn more about the spirit of life and being very receptive to the greater life around me. The animals must have sensed the energy radiating from me and wanted to be a part of it. I was delighted to be part of their lives.

The great psychologist of the last century, Abraham Maslow, suggested that we identify our peak moments and re-live them regularly to remind us what is possible. In the process of doing so we strengthen and stabilize our ability to re-connect to the source of life and increase the capacity to bring it down to where it can be used. These connections feed us, inspire us and lead us to the next challenge and opportunity to let our light shine. Our extraordinary experiences with nature, its plants and animal companions should be on the list of peak events to ponder. They draw us closer to the source of healing.

Invoking Nature's Energy For Healing

We are all part of a larger life. Our nature experiences are one of the ways of remembering and nourishing this connection. It is vital that we do so because it adds fresh energy, new outlooks and a vast ocean of nurturing interactions. In nature are many lessons of patience as life grows slowly in spite of many obstacles of drought, flood and cold. With patience we find persistence and perseverance for the most troublesome of times.

There are abundant signs of renewal in nature in spite of obvious obstacles. I remember walking in a small cave with my son one day. Deep in the cave we saw small plants growing in the dark because of a little earth and a growing seed even though without sunlight. Coming out of the cave we then noticed a tree nearby growing around an immense boulder; it was in the way but not enough to keep it from growing. Nearby were flower absorbing nutrients.

Each of these struggles are a metaphor for the healing we need medically and psychologically. There is gentleness in the softness of new grass. There is strength in the power of the wind and driving rain of thunderstorms. We can learn from the persistence of a tree to grow with a boulder in its path. It is like having an illness and a parent or spouse or sibling that is highly critical or neglectful. We can learn from the patience of a fragile flower stem pushing its way through the soil toward the sun. It is like a timid soul searching for its way without seeing the light to show the way. Nature is full of the strengths of healing energies eager to share its lessons learned over eons of time.

All of our experiences with nature are available to the creative imagination. When I lead a patient though a relaxation exercise I offer a few suggestions for how to invoke the nurturing, healing power of Mother Nature. These are the steps I have found helpful.

1. Relax comfortably.
2. Recall a pleasant memory in nature, an enjoyable experience of a favorite place on vacation, a hike in the woods, gorgeous view from a hill or the familiar backyard with its own aura of peacefulness. Each of these is a microcosm of a larger whole.
3. Open the mind's eye to this memory as a place that is safe and secure. Picture yourself there. Allow the experience to unfold. Smell the freshness of nature's vibrancy. Feel the pulsing presence of life in the grass, plants, trees, animals and people.
4. Look for a place to recline knowing that it is appropriate, safe and secure to do so.
5. Ask the higher self to move the attention from the physical body to the higher energies of heart-felt kindness, gentleness and beauty of nature's abundant healing energy.
6. Engage the mind by asking why it is necessary to be well (the obvious reasons need to be stated), why you deserve to be well (this conviction

lifts us above remorse and resentments) and what you will do with the healing received (practical ways you will add to the life of those around you).

7. Invite the energies of nature to flow through the top of the head down the spine through each of the nerves to muscles, joints, tendons and connecting tissues. Feel it improve the circulation where most needed, soothing, comforting and healing as it moves to each organ and cell of the body.
8. Soak it up, appreciating its source and the ability to be in tune with it. Enjoy the body's ability to be made whole, more healthy, and renewed in important ways.
9. Do this often and regularly until feeling the Oneness that has always been there and continues to expand in us and through us.

We are each a child of nature, cared for, watched over and nurtured until we can consciously become a center of healing energy. We are designed to be an active agent of nature's healing power to ourselves and those we serve.

Chapter 23

Seeing the End as a New Beginning

Death is a transition from this life to the next one. As a physician I have faced death closely with many patients and family members. I have been present with many during and soon after the passing. I have come to know that life continues without the physical body. After we leave the physical body our subconscious mind becomes our new conscious mind with all its fears and failures, hopes and successes, loves and delights. Most of all we become engaged in a vast new range of opportunity to grow, to learn and to serve on a grander scale.

This may sound strange to some but only because many of us over-identify with the physical body as the only sign of reality. There are a wide range of experiences that occur that verify these statements. However it often requires a personal experience to know for sure.

One of my earliest experiences of dying came during the medical training years. My patient was a woman in her 80s dying of congestive heart failure. Near the end of my visit with her one morning in the hospital I sat down near her and asked if she remembered any dreams recently. She looked at me in almost horror. With reassurance of my genuine interest, in a low voice, she said she did but that they bothered her a great deal. As we talked it became apparent that she did not routinely remember her dreams nor learn how to extract meaning from them. However, over the last few weeks she was dreaming of people close to her who had passed on. She thought they were nightmares because the people in them were dead. When I asked her to describe what was happening she said that they talked with her. They talked about how they were doing and how she was doing. It was an ordinary conversation that was very similar to what she would have with them when they were living.

I reassured her that they were there to help and were preparing her for where she would be going soon. They would be her tour guides. It is like taking a trip to another city or going on vacation except that we stay longer. The only thing we leave behind is our body and the stuff and things of physical life. We take everything else with us - our usual states of feeling, issues of concern, worries, fears, regrets and enjoyments. We take our assumptions of how we have done with our life, our unresolved disappointments, missed opportunities and all the memories of being loved and loving others. All the peaks and valleys go with us. With the uplift of our peaks and our accomplishments we receive impetus to heal the shadows and losses. We return to our real home.

In the 1970s I remember when Dr. Elizabeth Kubler-Ross began to talk about facing death with dignity. She described the difficulty of people facing death, the denial, frustration, depression, anger and finally acceptance. She saw patients successfully accept the fact of their pending deaths and sought to have more people reach the contentment that such a state brings. Although the medical community was in denial the public was interested and responded. Eventually she developed guidelines for how to approach death and dying which became known as the five stages of facing death. It became a more direct effort to help those approaching the transition we call death and has been used successfully by many.

Several years later, Dr. Ray Moody published his book, *Life After Life,* in which he carefully studied those with near-death experiences (NDEs). He found patterns to the reports of these events such as the rising out of the body, looking down upon the physical body and the activities of those around it, seeing a tunnel with a light at the end, reaching the end of it and being in the presence of a friend or someone very special. Dr. Moody legitimized the study of such events and inspired much further research. He reached the point where he began to teach people how to contact those who have passed on through the use of intense one-on-one sessions. He continues to speak and inspire researchers to explore this vital part of our lives, the continuity of life.

Near Death Experiences

A patient of mine recently reported this kind of experience: "It was 15 or so years ago. I was depressed over the break-up with my fiancée. I was clean and sober at the time. I do not remember the exact circumstances that brought on the 'near death experience'. I had considered suicide but did not attempt it. I suddenly saw this very bright light and indescribable warmth of love and peace. I was with all of my loved ones and friends that had passed on. It was the most wonderful and indescribable experience of my life. And since then I have not been afraid of death. I look forward to it! I am from a religious family but I do not practice any particular faith. I do believe in a God."

At times a major trauma invokes the presence of the soul. The soul has an agenda that it wants to accomplish. If it must manifest during a difficult time it may do so. It should also be considered a success not to ever need the soul to save us from our distress.

The latest research is being done by Jeff Long, M.D., a radiation oncologist who has been studying NDEs for several years. In the 1990s he created a web site for those who have experienced an NDE. Over time he accumulated over 5,000 episodes, approximately 700 of whom filled out a questionnaire he developed to explore people's experiences.

Based on these answers he was able to establish pattern percentages of common elements of the NDE. The most common defining aspect of an NDE is the out-of-body experience that is recorded by about 75%. A similar number notice an intense positive awareness of love, peace and beauty as well as heightened senses of alertness greater than in the fully wake state.

Hallucinatory experiences are much more often frightening and not peaceful in any way. Most NDErs are deeply affected by a brilliant light, more luminous but not hot, esoterically called the "cold light". Over half NDErs meet other beings, about 95% are deceased relatives with whom there is usually a very warm reception. Interestingly those who have passed over are also noted to be in a young state, at the peak of their recent physical life.

Approximately one-third with an NDE have a passing-through-a-tunnel experience, which is the awareness of consciousness moving from the body and brain to the emotion body. This is referred to by some as the 4th dimension when we are a point of consciousness with a 360-degree vision that also penetrates physical objects.

Only a small number have a life review. This is an additional profound experience of learning what is most important and what is not. To be shown our self-centeredness and selflessness is truly a divine gift that is life changing if taken to heart and adjustments are made. Of course, such an experience can be developed by persistent self-reflection and self-assessment by one so inclined without an NDE. However because few of us dig deep enough on our own for such an awareness, the life review is usually a profound event.

The most important and consistent result of having an NDE is the change in perspective of what is important and what is not. It becomes recognized to a high degree that how we treat one another is of great value. Loving-kindness and understanding really do make a difference. Most people's relationships distinctly improve. These are deeply healing and powerfully affect all those with whom we interact. There is often an increased degree of tolerance, willingness to forgive and genuine sense of goodwill.

Communicating With Those Who Pass

Over the last several years there has been growing interest in communicating with those who have passed on. John Edwards and James von Praag have both written several books on their abilities to intuitively communicate with those who have died. John had his own television program for a few years called "Crossing Over". James was a consultant for the television series "Ghost Whisperer," about a psychic who helps those who have recently deceased with unresolved problems. She helps them heal life issues and accept the final release "to the light." Now there is a reality show called "Monica the Medium" that is about a college student with the ability to communicate with those that have recently died. These mediums have a great deal to say about those who have passed on and yet continue to be in contact with us. I am convinced of their skill and dedication. They each have compelling stories that pass the tests of truth and integrity.

One of the best examples of communicating with a spirit is Olga Worrall. Trained as an elementary and secondary teacher she also had the ability to heal. With her husband, Ambrose she established a weekly healing session. One day a white-haired woman in a navy blue dress came and knelt at the altar before Olga. She had not seen her before and gently asked her, "What do you want me to pray for?" She looked up and said, "I don't know!" At that moment Olga perceived a man at her side, a spirit, who informed her, "I am her husband. I died last week. Tell her I am still with her and not to mourn for me." Olga leaned close to tell her what she saw and heard. The woman cried out, "My God, my God! I have been praying for some proof of my husband's survival. He died last week." A few weeks later she returned to thank Olga saying she now knows her husband lives. "He is with me", she said.

At the first American Holistic Medical Meeting in LaCrosse, WI, my brother attended Olga's healing lecture. He is a pediatrician from Duluth, MN. During the meeting he approached her for a possible healing of his migraine headaches. Before she worked on him she said, "We have some company here!" and went on to describe our dad who had recently passed over. In particular she said that he was wearing the most unusual hat. As she described it Jerry recognized it as dad's old hunting hat, well worn, with a few gorgeous pheasant feathers in the brim. My brother, the oldest of five, missed him the most. Her comments were very helpful to him and opened up the relationship with our dad in spirit that has grown over the years.

Rise Above The Narrow-Minded Authorities

All of these stories indicate the growing trend in the public to deal more directly with the continuity of life. As we accept this part of living we overcome the instinct to preserve life at all costs and the fear that all is lost when we die, that there is only a dark unknown. One of the saddest pending passings I witnessed involved an older man who was dying of cancer. When asked what he thought would happen after he passed he said, "I am not one of the chosen." He was a member of a church group that believes there are only a small number who will be taken to heaven after passing. I gave him reasons to not accept such a belief but I doubt it was enough to overcome the many years of brainwashing of his church.

What rubbish! What arrogance! We all live on. Our personality continues for a while until fully absorbed into the soul after which preparation is made for the next steps in growth and service. There is a great deal of variability. We all survive death and ultimately are drawn toward higher ways of being. We all move toward heaven eventually.

Although my experience with the clergy is limited what I have seen is that most are kind and concerned and yet know very little about the passing. They are generally compassionate and supportive and very helpful but not as reassuring as they could be with more open minds and better training.

Physicians in general are in a similar category. As a whole they are sensitive to the impact of the passing of a loved one on the individual as well as family and friends. However most seem very much unaware of what is to happen and unfortunately quite resistant to finding out. What their teachers do not teach them they do not believe or even explore, fortunately with a growing number of exceptions.

One friend of mine had a near death experience from a dye reaction injected into the spinal cord. Her head was tilted down instead of up, and the dye went around the lining of the brain instead of down the spinal cord. She rose out of her body into the ceiling where she observed and heard all that occurred. She heard the sharp sound of the EKG flat-lining, meaning that her heart stopped beating. When she returned to her body she remembered all that had happened. Who said what when and the multiple quick reactions resulting in her return to the body all registered quite clearly in her mind. Upon awaking she was excited about the experience and related the details to those present. The room of nurses and doctors was totally silent followed by an angry retort from one of the surgeons who then stomped out of the room. The other physician would not confirm publically what she said was true for several years.

There are many wonderful exceptions to this one. In her book, *Forever Ours*, Janis Amatuzio, M.D., relates the story of a woman in her 30s undergoing a thyroidectomy who had a cardiac arrest during surgery. The surgery team did everything they could for several minutes until it was clear there would be no response. As the head surgeon finally left the room he yelled out "I will not let this happen." He went back into the operating room, looked up at the ceiling and said, "Mary, Mary come back down here." He re-started resuscitation efforts and she recovered.

Death does not happen until the soul disconnects. It is not just a function of the heart and brain shutting down. There can be a more subtle level of life present that can be reawakened up to the point when the indwelling life leaves the body. The story of Lazarus is more than a myth. As long as the pilot light is on life can be re-awakened.

An Unexpected Death Does Not End

A few years ago a financial consultant heard the tragic news that his younger brother had died in a car accident. He took a few weeks off work to help his family and himself adjust to this sudden loss. Soon thereafter I had a chance to ask him if he had any dreams of his brother since the passing. He was surprised I asked and wasn't sure if an event that happened to him was relevant. He related a night experience that began with him "meeting my brother in a parking lot. I recognized him and expressed my delight to see him for the first time since his passing. My brother took me to a room where he was staying. It was in a large apartment complex. Inside his room the furniture, wall pictures and music were exactly as he had in his earthly home. The boom box was just like the one he had here and turned up loud as well. We chatted awhile and then began to wrestle like when we were young. In the midst of the wrestling I felt intensely close to my brother, knowing for sure this was him. I began to weep and quickly woke up."

A few weeks later he had a dream where he was at a picnic setting. His brother came up to him, thinned down. While living he ate well and exercised vigorously until the last few years before he died when he put on some weight. In the night experience he commented to his brother that he was slim now. His brother said he could be either way now, and promptly became larger and all buffed up.

My friend said that he rarely remembered his dreams and was not sure what it meant. I reassured him that this was more than a dream, that he had a visit with his brother. They were in contact in spirit and this would probably continue for some time. Then he related a dream that their youngest brother had soon after the accident. There were three boys in the family.

His youngest brother also had a nighttime experience. In this state he was visiting their mother in her house. The telephone rang. His mother answered it and said it was for him. The brother who had recently died was on the line and greeted him warmly. The youngest brother was perplexed, filled with questions about what happened, where he was, and how he was doing. He asked many questions. All the questions were answered to his satisfaction and he felt quite relieved as a result. He knew his brother had died of an overdose of drugs but wasn't sure if it was intentional or not. He found out from his deceased bother that it was not intentional and not due to street drugs being taken at the time. He admitted that he drank and took drugs excessively and that he was now getting the help he needed to understand and overcome these urges. He had recently been through financial difficulties leading to a divorce and severe depression.

These experiences are common. Approximately 70% of people say they have contact of some kind with a loved one who passes over. Whenever I give talks about this topic there are always a few who want to share their experience as well. Sharing can be healing. It is one of the ways we process the passing of an important friend or family member. It is very reassuring to those who recall such visits. There is an inner sense that it is just as real as the living person when in physical form. Continuity of life is experienced as a fact of life.

The Joy of Passing Over

My own father's passing was sudden and unexpected although providing me with an extraordinary experience. As this particular Labor Day approached I had an urge to visit my parents. Upon entering their home I was warmly greeted by my dad. We went into the living room and sat to chat. He began to talk at length about the value of love, how important it was in all aspects of life, especially family but also in work and in everything you do. He said that love does make the world go round, nurtures all relationships when given a chance and is the essence of all religious effort.

He continued on this theme for several minutes. I had never experienced him quite this way before. This was unusual to hear from him. Soon thereafter we moved onto other topics, watched the news and had our meals together. Over the weekend we played golf and had an unusually wonderful time together. Unusual for us also was that my mother was not home. She was visiting relatives several hundred miles away allowing just the two of us to have the time of our lives.

At the end of the weekend as I was preparing to leave he asked that I join him in hunting ducks later in the fall. I politely demurred knowing that I most likely would not. I had long lost interest in it though I have many warm memories of being with my dad and brothers for the annual fall hunt of pheasants and ducks. It was wonderful to hear his excitement when the northern flight was on route. This meant that the annual migration of geese from Canada was on its way to warmer climates during the winter months. And we might get a few delicious meals out of it.

Two months later, I received a call at about one AM. My older brother said, "There has been an accident. Dad has died." He and my older sister had been hunting with him for four days. As they would later recall, the sun was going down when one lone duck came flying over the decoy cluster. Dad took aim, fired and hit the bird. He was delighted to bag one more before the end of the day. They gathered up the decoys. As dad handed the last one to my sister he fell over. They made efforts to resuscitate him but he did not recover. My brother is a pediatrician and my sister a registered nurse. They knew what to do but it was not enough. His time had come.

After the call from my brother I made arrangements to fly home only a few hours later. Around 6 AM that morning while waiting at the small airport in LaCrosse, WI, I was pacing the waiting area, the only passenger scheduled for the quick flight to Minneapolis-St. Paul terminal. Suddenly I felt my dad's presence right next to me. He was happier than I had ever seen him. He highlighted the good he had done, the struggles he had overcome, and essentially the successes of his life, mainly raising a family of five children. He really was radiating joy, a wonderful sense of accomplishment and a deep sense of contentment. In the short time of his passing he realized what happened. He was enjoying the rewards of his persistent efforts to do the best he could with the life he had. He was thrilled with where he was. I was elated to share it with him.

As a result of this experience with him I had deeper appreciation for the life he led and how well he had done. He was raised in poverty in North Dakota. His father was a coal miner and contracted tuberculosis when a young man and was unable to support the family. He went to bed hungry many nights during the Depression years. He learned to hunt to put food on the table. With his passing there was no grief in me, though I participated in supporting my mother, sisters and brothers as best I could. Most of the family were glad to hear of his visit with me and found the experience very reassuring. Subsequently one brother and sister had several visits with him during the wake and sleep state. We are delighted and honored to continue our relationship with him.

Guidelines For Preparing To Die

Pending death and taking care of a loved one who is dying have their challenges. I have had family members and friends go through intense turmoil due to extended care in the final stages of dying. Fortunately there are a growing number of programs that offer a great deal of comfort, reassurance and practical advice in how to manage the final days. However the struggle is still overwhelming for many. As the body deteriorates there is a loss of the sense of time. Suffering occurs from pain, hunger, weakness and depression. The medical field is now much more supportive with the medication and services needed.

Ideally a team approach is best so that there is a rotation of duties allowing adequate sleep, nutrition and usual activities for those involved. When these are not present only the best can be done, and this must be accepted as reasonable to prevent guilt over not having done enough. Guidelines now include attention to the physical, psychological and spiritual realms.

Hospice has developed many ways to provide comfort and support for those approaching the passing. They should be called upon whenever possible. They provide professional nursing support for home care, medication usage and effective counseling. Hospice also trains a large number of volunteers, many of whom become angels of compassion and cheerfulness to those involved in the transition process. They are well trained to provide basic psychological support for the patient and the family. But they do not become involved until the last six months of life.

Palliative Care is a new medical specialty providing professional guidance for comprehensive end of life care. Directed by a physician the team consists of nurses and other medical personnel that may also involve Hospice. Usually the care is provided in the hospital although it often continues in the home. Palliative care is designed to reduce suffering and improve quality of life for those with advanced disease regardless of the stage. The psychological and spiritual needs are comprehensively addressed as well with advance disease near the end of life.

Based on these stories and my own experiences I offer these suggestions for those preparing to die.

1. Engage medical and hospice services to the degree needed and available. Medication can relieve discomfort and ensure sleep for the one who is ill.

2. Ensure basic home health care for the patient, and sleep and break time for family, friends and neighbors involved.
3. Consider the frequent use of favorite music, the reading of favorite stories and reviewing enjoyable memories.
4. Recall the best expressions of love, loving service to others and any expressions of kindness or understanding.
5. Review work left undone, unresolved fears, worries and errors using forgiveness freely as willing and able.
6. Encourage discussions of purposes of living, what lies ahead and the role of spirit depending on the interest of those involved.

The end of life is a unique opportunity to care for the loved one who is passing. With the right perspective and support, this can be a very rewarding and inspiring experience for all involved. However it can also be very tiring and depressing. If resentment begins to grow from fatigue and frustration, professional help should be sought as soon as possible. The time of transition can and should be a celebration of the good well done drawing upon all the resources available.

Healing From The Loss Of Those We Love

Many do not work through the relationship with the loved one who passes. I hear it often in the office. Unspoken frustration and lack of communication is far too common. However, it is never too late to do more. We always have a chance to work through our relationships even after a passing. It is best to do so while alive but often not possible especially with aging parents and those who have moved away. With a sincere effort we can initiate healing at any time. All healing occurs within. It can be aided with an awareness that the one who has passed is still accessible in our heart and mind.

Writing a good-bye letter is often effective. The unresolved issues are important to clarify, especially with an honest expression of deep feelings and thoughts about what happened, what did not happen and how you would have liked things to have worked out better. Offering forgiveness, expressing forgiveness and proclaiming love for the good that is present will invoke healing. Whether the person is present or not, a genuine effort to resolve differences invokes the power of healing.

For some it is very helpful to listen carefully for unusual dream activity. The dreams may not be the common psychological processing but an actual contact with the individual who has passed and others who may be present with them. Many report such an experience as another chance to talk things over or at least confirm a dedicated love for each other. When this occurs it can be very healing.

The passing from this life to the next is a transition from one set of activities to another. Only the physical plane changes, not the emotions, mind or spirit. It is similar to other transitions in life, like graduating from grade school, high school or college. It is like moving from single life to marriage and then having a child. It is like changing from one kind of career to the next. These are all transitions in which we take our feelings, thoughts and aspirations with us. These change as we review what happened, extract meaning from all the events of our life and aspire to do more.

Soon after passing many other activities are set in motion. Those who report near death experiences often recount a life review. In this way we see the way we choose to act, interact and react to life's circumstances. There is always help available. The soul is in charge. We learn who we have been. We learn that we really are a center of love, wisdom and joy. We learn how to grow into our destiny.

Embrace The Continuity Of Life

Eventually we will embrace the continuation of living like we do the seasons of the year: spring, summer, fall and winter, and its correlates of life, death, after-life and re-birth. My hope is that this philosophy will help confront the skepticism rampant in the public and the medical community about the continuity of life. We do live on. Medical research is expanding and will help us provide much greater support in the near future.

The reasons to pursue study in the continuity of life is that it has many healing benefits to individuals, families and society. There is still tremendous fear associated with dying. The reasons for fear are numerous and include the fear of losing family and close friends forever, that once the body dies the relationship is over. There is fear of suffering while we die. There is fear that life has little meaning if it is all over when we die. None of these are true.

Doctors are encouraged now to provide the medications needed for comfort for those who are dying. Life has meaning especially near the end when we are given opportunities to heal old wounds. Those who confront their past not only diminish suffering but at times heal physically. Meaning is increased for those who choose to pursue it. Our relationships continue though at a less conscious level. Many who pass over continue supporting, nurturing, watching and enjoying us for an extended period of time. Being receptive to possible connections with those who have passed over can mobilize healing at a deep level.

Summary Comments

Chapter 24

How to Mobilize Your Healing Power

Learning and doing are two different steps. The obvious examples include learning to drive and doing it well, learning how to speak in front of a group and doing it well, and having children and raising them well. We can read all about it. Hear people tell us how it is done. But at some point we have to get behind the wheel, get in front of a group and change the diapers ourselves.

The same principle applies to health and healing. Learning what to eat, how much to exercise, why to forgive, what to think and how to meditate are only first steps. Then we must implement them so they take hold and become part of our lifestyle.

The two main obstacles for succeeding are the power of the past and the power of the moment. There are many obstacles to healing and wholeness. Overcoming the obvious ones of the past and present will provide energy and insight for the others. Most of all, overcoming obstacles provides the means to energize what we seek to build and bring to blossom in our life.

The power of the past is the momentum of familiarity. *One in the hand is better than two in the bush* is the old saying. This is means that what we have should be appreciated more than what we may receive. However, clinging to what we have may limit what is possible to learn, grow and develop. The past is an obstacle if we use it as the only guideline for deciding the future. It can become a force of inertia that ingrains our less than optimal habits of eating, exercising and all kinds of activities.

When it comes to establishing new habits of any kind we meet the bodyguards of the past. These are the familiar ways and habits of how we pursue the day, consider our major relationships, react to criticism, and respond to new opportunity. These bodyguards of the past are powerful influences that maintain the status quo and make it hard to change, even when we are convinced of the need to do so. When we empower them through fear, doubt and anger, they become formidable forces that resist change, necessary insight and healing.

We rise above the past by accepting the truth of what has happened and learning all we can from it. Accepting the truth means forgiving ourself for the failure to do better and not knowing the consequences of our behavior. "I accept who I am, who I've been and who I am growing to be" begins the process. The complexities of emotions, people and events do not heal easily but do with persistence and patience. As we heal the past we marshal the energies connected with it to propel us forward.

The other main obstacle to applying what we learn is the power of the present. We are strongly influenced by how we feel and the need for comfort. An old wise friend often reminded me of this challenge when he would ask "Do you want to be comfortable or do you want to change?" Creating new habits of action, feeling and thought have an effect on our priorities. The priorities of thinking and feeling are based on expectations of self-satisfaction and self-serving ways. Comfort and pleasure are strong present priorities. These must be confronted to establish new ways of solving problems and setting goals. We confront them by committing ourself to our primary priorities and intensely pursing them.

If the present is largely filled with regrets and remorse it will limit our ability to heal and be healthy. You can't appreciate what you do have if you only think of what you don't have. If negative experiences dominate our attention it is harder to be aware of and receptive to new options and new habits for transforming change. The present must be positive.

Mobilizing the power of healing depends on three major choices: clarifying what needs to be healed, identifying the resources available for healing, and integrating the new effort into the fabric of the day.

1. Clarify the present need carefully. Clarifying the need of the moment is a little more complicated than it first appears. There is often a strong impulse to focus on what we do not want in terms of pain, limited movement and whatever is unpleasant. If the problem is a physical ailment or disease we often just want to get rid of the pain, illness or fear of it.

However we are far more likely to heal by finding the risk factors that preceded it and diminishing those. The risk factors involve the choices made that set in motion the problem: choices of convenience, ignoring warning signs and failing to connect the dots. The real needs are how to mobilize compassion, courage and cheerfulness.

Compassion is a genuine need. We need a deep sense of caring for all those involved in the issue including ourself. Compassion engages a sense of the suffering and the need for forgiveness for ourselves and others. Compassion mobilizes a serious dedication to be a loving presence no matter the circumstance or person involved. It awakens the mind to look for ways to be helpful and useful. If this were present in the first place in greater amounts, how much better would we respond to a new problem?

Courage is the strength that helps us confront problems directly and quickly. Not all problems of disagreement, unfairness or abuse can be confronted immediately. Many times we are in an inferior position as a child or employee needing the job or overly dependent on the group to which we belong and fearful of challenging it. The energy of courage compels us to speak up if only to ask questions to find out more, to uncover basic motivations or identify self-serving intentions. Courage can also help us connect to overlying purposes and assumed agreements of engagement. If courage were sufficiently available when the problem arose, how differently would we respond to a new crisis?

Cheerfulness is enjoyment of the moment. More than a funny story it is a sense of lightheartedness when someone has done something odd, silly or too seriously. In retrospect it is often easy to see the crazy predicaments we set in motion by our attachments to small-minded wishes and wants. Cheerfulness enables a detached view and a sense of optimism, that whatever the problem we are confident in our ability to rise above it and be better because of the challenge of it. It helps us move from the serious to the sublime. How much suffering would we prevent by being more cheerful when the problem first appears knowing there are ways through it?

What often needs to be healed is activating what is missing. If this strength were present how much better would have been the response? The real need to be healed is awakening the virtue most missing and most needed at this time. Is it calmness, confidence, acceptance and forgiveness, or strength, resilience, dedication, directness and dignity?

2. Identify the resources available. The resources reside within our own set of experiences and the spirit within. Resources also reside within the relationships of family, friends and co-workers. As we pay attention to what happens to us we create a database of events, feelings and ideas. We each have a rich heritage of what has happened and why. We have learned in many ways the consequences of the choices made. The laws of living reveal themselves as we see the patterns over time. These can be reviewed and reflected upon for self-renewal. In particular our resources include patience, persistence and initiative.

If the need is patience, we look for memories of having been patient in difficult situations. We consider examples of patience in nature such as the movements of the seasons where new growth always gives way to blossoms and fruit. The flowers and trees surrender to a loss of vitality and a winter of withdrawal to be later reborn and regenerated. For every winter there is a spring, for every spring a summer, and for every summer a fall. The mastery of patience not only helps us overcome obstacles but helps us find companions that can help us complete our major missions. We can do this by recalling people in our life who confronted crises by being calm and thoughtful rather than rash and impulsive. The power in patience is that it leads to a greater sense of the purpose of the larger presence of which we are a part.

If we need persistence, the resources for finding it are in the lives of those we know who have overcome an immense challenge with an

illness or tragedy. We find it when we review our own rise from childhood to adulthood to self-sufficiency to form our own families with children and friends. Persistence is present in great figures when we consider the fortitude of Churchill to protect England or Mother Theresa to serve the endless number dying in the streets of Calcutta. Or the wonderful example of Harry Potter seemingly overwhelmed by the early loss of his parents, the disdain of his adopted family and cruelty of fellow students. If they can survive that surely I can handle this. Of course, the real heroes of persistence not only survive but also thrive. They dedicate themselves to the mission of adding something of value to the turmoil they confront in spite of the obstacles present.

If we need more initiative, we look back to when we made big decisions. The best decisions we make in our life are the turning points, the peak events of initiating new direction. We chose new directions when we chose a new job, worked our way upward to more responsible positions and accepted greater responsibility. We chose new directions when we found a mate with whom to commit ourselves and start a family. We chose a new direction when we found a new place to live or moved to a new city. We made a big decision when we joined a new group with which to study or pursue a particular issue in art, music, meditation or volunteer service. All of these are events of taking the bull by the horns and choosing a new direction. The more initiative we develop the more likely we will confront issues directly as they arise. The more we confront issues directly the more we prevent disease from continual worry or deterioration from neglect and apathy.

3. Integrate the chosen changes into the day. Apply what you learn and admire in others. Until new habits are performed regularly they do not stick. Until new ways of thinking, feeling and acting are repeated over and over they do not become dominant in our life. The goal is to have the best attitude, the best frame of mind and the greatest compelling urge to heal and grow in charge. Otherwise the lower urges and instincts take over. The shadow side of old habits keep us bound down to limited options and limited chances for healing.

The way we integrate our new intentions for change begin with how we start the day. If we begin the day by remembering the new resolutions, they will be more with us throughout the day. Even only a few minutes of reflection awakens our interest and inspiration for change. During brief intervals of the day we can recall our new emphasis and consider how to feel and act with the new set of beliefs we are seeking to install. This is the opposite of reawakening misery memories that build reservoirs of distress and despair. What is exercised grows. We reap what we sow. Sow the best seeds of thought and feeling and we bring to blossom a harvest of beauty and abundance.

Midday is also an ideal time to remember to integrate new efforts. I am a big fan of after-lunch naps. It is an excellent time to rest the body and enhance digestion. Most of all midday is a time to review what happened in the early part of the day. How well did things go? How could I have made them better? What did I miss? What did I enjoy? What did I learn? A brief rest time for the body is good for the heart and mind to re-connect with the higher aspirations we are creating. In a quiet time we can also prepare for what is to come with eager expectation of something interesting and enjoyable.

The main goal is to create a new identity of who we are. In the past we may have created an identity of problems, illness or injury. New intentions for healing require a full commitment, a new self. One of the old ways of creating a new self is to choose a new mission. In religious and some psychology circles a new name is actually chosen. In positions of higher authority a new title is conferred. Some companies go to great length to have a respectful title for every position.

In healing it may be helpful to create a new affirmation that synthesizes the changes desired. It is helpful to create a phrase that easily summarizes the new goal and mission. Examples may be:

> "I have come here to be more loving, kind, courageous and consistent."
> "I have come here to be more forgiving and tolerant, more willing to see other points of view."
> "It is easy to accept my past, the good I have learned and the good yet to do."

"It is easy to look forward to the future and my ability to grow and learn."

"I am strong, resilient and persistent."

"I am a child of God eager to fulfill my destiny and determined to do so."

Of course, having an affirmation and living it are two different things. We energize our affirmation with the higher self. The power source is our higher self. As we cooperate with it, invite its involvement and honor its presence, it works its way through us. We make the connection with a sincere appeal to its guidance. As we recall prior peak events we re-energize its presence within us. As we re-dedicate ourselves to its agenda we open our awareness to its impact upon us and through us. The value of the affirmation is that it becomes a focal point through which the higher self can work its way through us for the healing needed.

We are each part of the larger life in which we live and move and have our being. As we contribute to the smaller world in which we live we add to the whole and more is revealed to us. The more we devote to improving the lives of those with whom we live, the more we contribute to the larger life. As we do our part we develop greater eyes to see and ears to hear. We increase our awareness of the abundance of love, wisdom, joy and healing energy. The greater connection we create to the whole and its missions the more its healing power can flow to us and through us. This is how we mobilize our healing power.

A Prayer to Mobilize Healing Power

May the divine source within me be present now. I am one with my source of love, wisdom and joy. I am ready to accept the missions of this day.

Help me to call forth the strength of my soul, eager to express what I have to offer. Show me how to confront fear, doubt, and worry. Show me how to confront the past, as I grasp the lessons that have been learned. Help me to rise above the ashes of guilt, frustration, anger and impatience to make room for the caring, confidence and courage that is my true nature.

My needs are to face the responsibilities of this day, the people I meet, the past that I carry and the events that unfold. I need your help to remind me of my true needs and what I have come here to be.

Help me to look forward to the routines of this day. To infuse them with a fresh feeling of enthusiasm and optimism. Help me to know of what I am capable, the resources available, and the strengths that I have. Awaken me to the patience and persistence that is present now.

Open my eyes to see the beauty that is in front of me, to see the intentions of others to do the right thing in the right way, and to see when this is not so in myself and others.

Open my ears to hear the quiet beauties of nature, the enjoyable sounds of family, friends and healing music. Help me to hear the pleas for attention within myself, and how to heal and harmonize them. Help me to hear the meanings behind the words of those I meet, and respond to the highest extent possible.

Use these hands to serve those that I can with what I have to offer. Use me as an agent of goodwill and generosity to each of those I meet and think about this day. Help me to make a difference this day.

I am grateful for all that I receive in kindness, reassurance and compassion. I honor the good that is present within and around me. I am healing, whole and healthy in every way! I am loving, wise, strong and joyful in all that I do!

END NOTES

Chapter 1. Causes of disease are not mysteries. Page 10

1. Bland, Jeff, Ph.D. *Genetic Nutritioneering*, McGraw-Hill, 1999.
2. Bland, Jeff, Ph.D. *The Disease Delusion: Conquering the Causes of Chronic Illness for a Healthier, Longer and Happier Life.* HarperCollins, 2014.
3. Fu, Ping. *Bend, Not Break - A Life in Two Worlds.* Portfolio/Penguin, 2012.
4. Leichtman, Robert, M.D. *Psychic Vandalism and Preventing It From Ruining Our Lives.* Enthea Press, 2008.
5. Norling, Sharon, M.D., MPH. *Your Doctor is Wrong - Survival Guide for Dismissed, Misdiagnosed or Mistreated.* Morgan James Publishing, 2014.
6. Myss, Caroline. *Why People Don't Heal and How They Can.* Three Rivers Press, 1997.
7. Seligman, Martin, Ph. D. *Learned Pessimism.* First Vintage Books, 1990.
8. Shealy, C. Norman, M.D., Ph.D. *The Pain Game.* Celestial Arts, 1976.

Chapter 2. Activate practical principles of healing. Page 19

1. Adams, Marilee G., Ph. D. *Change Your Questions Change Your Life.* Berritt Kohler, 2004.
2. Bailey, Alice A. *Esoteric Healing.* Lucis Publishing Co., 1953.
3. Keller, Helen. *Optimism.* Enthea Press, 1903.
4. Leichtman, Robert, M.D. *Psychic Self Destruction and How to Reverse It.* Enthea Press, 2012.
   Lincoln-Bradley Publishing Group, 1996.
5. Leichtman, Robert, M.D., & Carl Japikse. *The Way to Health.* Ariel Press, 1979.

6. Schlessinger, Dr. Laura. *Bad Childhood Good Life.* HarperCollins, 2006.
7. Seligman, Martin, Ph. D. *Flourish.* Free Press, 2011.
8. Shealy, C. Norman, M.D., Ph.D. *Life Beyond 100 - Secrets of the Fountain of Youth.* Tarcher/Penguin, 2005.
9. Sinatra, Steven. *Optimum Health - A Natural Lifesaving Prescription for Your Body and Mind.*
10. Tavris, Janet. *Anger: The Misunderstood Emotion.* Touchstone, 1984.
11. 11. Warren, Rick. *The Purpose Driven Life.* Zondervan, 2002.

REGENERATE PHYSICAL WELLBEING

Chapter 3. Five steps to diet dynamism. Page 28

1. Gaby, Alan, M.D. *Nutritional Medicine Textbook.* Goodwill Books, 2010.
2. Campbell, T. Colin, Ph. D. & Thomas Campbell. *The China Study.* Benbella, 2004.
3. Ornish, Dean, M.D. *The Spectrum - A Scientifically Proven Program to Feel Better, Live Longer, Lose weight, Gain Health.* Ballantine Books, 2007.
4. Reilly, Mikki. *Your Primal Body - The Paleo Way to Living Lean, Fit, and Healthy at Any Age.* Lifelong Books, 2013.
5. Shealy, C. Norman, M.D., Ph.D. *90 Days to Self-Health.* The Dial Press, 1978
6. Smith, Pamela, M.D., M.P.H. *Demystifying Weight Loss.* Healthy Living Books, 2007.
7. Willett, Walter C., M.D. *Eat, Drink, and Be Healthy - The Harvard Medical School Guide to Healthy Eating.* Free Press, 2001.

Chapter 4. How to re-vitalize with exercise. Page 38

1. Cooper, Kenneth, M.D., M.P.H. *Aerobics.* Bantam Book, 1968.
2. Cooper, Kenneth, M.D., M.P.H. *Aerobics for Women.* Bantam Book, 1973.
3. Crowley, C. & Lodge, H., M.D. *Younger Next Year - The Exercise Program.* Workman Publishing Co., 2016.

3. Radha. Swami Sivinanda. *Kundalini Yoga*. Barnes & Noble, 1999.
4. Stearn, Jess. *Youth, Yoga & Reincarnation*. Market Paperback, 1969.

Chapter 5. Serene sleep strategies. Page 47

1. Davis, M., Ph.D., Eshelman, E., MSW, M. McKay, Ph. D. *The Relaxation and Stress Reduction Workbook*. New Harbinger Publications, 2008.
2. Dement, William, M.D. & Vaughan, C.C. *The Promise of Sleep*. Delacorte Press, 1999.
3. Schultz and Luthe. *Autogenic Training*. 1932.

Chapter 6. How to find the harmony of hormone balance. Page 52

1. Ahlgrimm, Marla and Kells, John. *The HRT Solution*. Avery, 2003.
2. Crisler, Dr. John. *Testosterone Replacement Therapy - A Recipe for Success*. www.AllThingsMale.com, 2014.
3. Kime, Zane. *Sunlight Could Save Your Life*. World Health Publications, 1980.
4. Kohlstadt, Ingrid. *Food and Nutrition in Disease Management*. CRC Press, 2009.
5. Lee, John, M.D. & Hopkins, V. *Dr. John Lee's Hormone Balance Made Simple*. Warner Wellness, 2006.
6. Lundin, Mia, R.N., N.P. *Female Brain Gone Insane*. Health Communications, 2009.
7. Morgenthaler, Abraham, M.D. *The Truth About Men and Sex*. Henry Holt, 2015.
8. Regelson, William, M.D., and Colman, Carol. *The Super Hormone Promise - Nature's Antidote to Aging*. Simon and Schuster, 1996.
9. Smith, Pamela, M.D., MPH. *Women's Hormones - Your Guide to Natural Hormone Treatments for PMS, Menopause, Osteoporosis, PCOS and More*. Square One Publishers, 2010.
10. Wright, Jonathan, M.D. & Morgenthaler, John. *Natural Hormone Replacement - For Women Over 45*. Smart Publications, 1997.

Chapter 7. Healing pain leads to wholeness. Page 69

1. Helms, Joe, M.D. *Acupuncture Energetics- A Clinical Approach for Physicians, 1995.*
2. Jemmett, Rick, B.Sc (PT). *Spinal Stabilization - The New Science of Back Pain.* Lilbris Hubris Publishing, 2013.
3. Johnson, Jim, P.T. *The Multifidus Back Pain Solution - Simple Exercises That Target the Muscles That Count.* New Harbinger Publications, 2002.
4. Melzack, Ronald. *The Puzzle of Pain.* Basic Books, 1974.
5. C. Shealy, Norman, M.D. *The Pain Game.* Celestial Arts, 1976.

Chapter 8. Sources of energy are everywhere. Page 77

1. Baraz, James & Alexander, Shoshana. *Awakening Joy - 10 Steps to Happiness.* Parallax Press, 2012.
2. Karagulla, Shafica, M.D. & Dora van Gelder Kunz. *The Chakras and the Human Energy Fields.* Quest Books, 1989.
3. Leichtman, Robert, M.D. *Faith Fatigue.* Enthea Press, 2001.
4. Losada, M. & Heaphy, E. "The role of positivity and connectivity in the performance of business teams: A nonlinear dynamics model." *American Behavioral Scientist*, 47(6), 740-765, 2004.
5. Lyubomirsky, Sonja. *The How of Happiness.* Penguin Press, 2007.
6. Perlmutter, David, M.D. *The Better Brain Book.* Riverhead Books, 2004.
7. Somers, Suzanne. *Ageless: The Naked Truth About Bioidentical Hormones.* Random House LLC.
8. Teitelbaum, Jacob, M.D. *From Fatigued to Fantastic.* Penguin Group, 2007.
9. Weatherby, Dr. Dicken. *Naturally Raising Your HGH Levels.* Bear Mountain Publishing, 2005.

EXPRESS LOVING KINDNESS AND UNDERSTANDING
Chapter 9. Transform stress to stimulate healing. Page 89

1. Childre, Doc & Rozman, Deborah, Ph.D. *Transforming Stress - The HeartMath Solution for Relieving Worry, Fatigue, and Tension.* New Harbinger Publications, 2005.
2. Green, Elmer & Alyce. *Beyond Biofeedback.* Knoll Publishing Co., 1989.
3. Maslow, Abraham. *Toward a Psychology of Being.* Sublime Books, 2014.
4. Selye, Hans. *The Stress of Life.* McGraw-Hill, 1956.
5. Shealy, C. Norman, M.D., Ph.D. *90 Days to Self-Health - Biogenics: How to Control All Types of Stress by Yourself Through a Complete Health Program of Autogenics, Diet, Vitamins and Exercise.* The Dial Press, 1976.

Chapter 10. How to be relaxed, calm and confident. Page 98

1. Benson, Herb, M.D. *The Relaxation Response.* HarperCollins, 1975.
2. Davis, Martha, & Eshelman, Elizabeth. *The Relaxation & Stress Reduction Workbook.* New Harbinger Publications, 2008.
3. Hartley, Elda. *Biofeedback: Yoga of the West.* Hartley Film, 1976.
4. Kermani, Dr, Kai. *Autogenic Training - The Effective Way to Holistic Health.* Souvenir Press, 2010.

Chapter 11. Relationships generate growth and self renewal. Page 105

1. Gottman, John & Silver, Nan. *The Seven Principles for Making Marriage Work.* Weidenfeld & Nicolson, 1999
2. Miller, John G. *QBQ: The Question Behind the Question - What to Really Ask Yourself to Eliminate Blame, Victim Thinking, Complaining and Procrastination.* G.P. Putnams Sons, 2001.

3. Leichtman, Robert R., M.D. & Carl Japikse. *Healing Emotional Wounds*. Enthea Press, 1979.
4. Pecci, Ernest F., M.D. *Rise Above It - A Psychiatrist Looks Within for a Higher Meaning to Life*. Pavior, 2005.
5. Schlessinger, Dr. Laura. *The Proper Care and Feeding of Marriage*. HarperCollins, 2007.
6. Sheindlin, Judge Judy. *Keep It Simple, Stupid You're Smarter Than You Look - Uncomplicating Families in Complicated Times*. HarperCollins, 2000.

Chapter 12. How to expose and expel resistance to healing. Page 116

1. Leichtman, Robert R., M.D. *Psychic Self-Destruction & How to Reverse It*. Enthea Press, 2012.
2. Leichtman, Robert R., M.D. *Psychic Vandalism*. Enthea Press, 2008.
3. Myss, Carolyn. *Why People Don't Heal and How They Can - A Practical Programme for Healing Body, Mind and Spirit*. Bantam Books, 1998.
4. Norling, Sharon. M.D. *Your Doctor is Wrong*. Morgan James Publishing, 2014.
5. Seligman, Martin, Ph.D. *Flouirish - A Visionary New Understanding of Happiness and Well-being*. Free Press, 2012.
6. Seligman, Martin. *Learned Optimism - How to Change Your Mind and Your Life*. Vintage, 2006.
7. Simmons, Gary. *The I of the Storm - Embracing Conflict, Creating Peace*. Unity Books, 2001.
8. Tavris, Janet. *Anger: The Misunderstood Emotion*. Touchstone, 1984.

Chapter 13. The healing energy of work well done. Page 123

1. Anders, George. *The Rare Find - How Great Talent Stands Out*. Portfolio/Penguin, 2011.
2. Besant, Annie and Leadbeater, C. *Creating Character*. The Theosophical Publishing House, 1951.

3. Canfield, Jack. *The Success Principles - How to Get From Where You Are to Where You Want to Be.* Harper Collins, 2005.
4. Evans, Harold. *They Made America - From the Steam Engine to the Search Engine.* Little, Brown, 2004.
5. Geilan, Michelle. *Broadcasting Happiness - The Science of Igniting and Sustaining Positive Change.* BenBella Books, 2015.
6. Patterson, James. *Making Your Career Meaningful: A Practical Toolbox.* Amazon, 2015.
7. Rohr, Richard. *Falling Upward - A Spirituality for the Two Halves of Life.* Jossey-Bass, 2011.

AWAKEN THE GENIUS WITHIN
Chapter 14 Restore the magic of memory. Page 129

1. Braverman, Eric R., M.D. *The Healing Nutrients Within - How to Use Amino Acids to Achieve Optimum Health.* Keats Publishing, 1997.
2. Dean, Ward, Morgenthaler, John, Fowkes, S.W. *Smart Drugs II: The Next Generation.* Smart Publications, 1994
3. Green, Elmer, Ph.D. *The Ozawkie Book of the Dead - Alzheimer's Isn't What You Think It Is.* Philosophical Research Society, Inc., 2001
4. Hyman, Mark, M.D. *The UltraMind Solution - Fix Your Broken Brain by Healing Your Body First.* Scribner, 2009.
5. Memory. *National Geographic*, November, 2007.
6. Morgenthaler, John. *Smart Drugs & Nutrients.* Ward Dean, Smart Publication, 1991.
7. Leichtman, Robert, M.D. & Japikse, Carl. *The Art of Living: The Mind and Its Uses.* Ariel Press, 1978.
8. Perlmutter, David, M.D. *The Better Brain Book.* The Berkeley Publishing Group, 2004.
9. Perlmutter, David, M.D. *Grain Brain: The Surprising Truth About Wheat, Carbs and Sugar - Your Brain's Silent Killers.* Little, Brown and Co., 2013.

Chapter 15. How to discover and develop intuition. Page 139

1. Bailey, Alice A. *From Intellect to Intuition*. Lucis Press, 1932.
2. Dossey, Larry, M.D. *The Power of Premonitions - How Knowing the Future Can Shape Our Lives.* Cutton, 2009.
3. Leadbeater, Charles. *The Inner Life*. A Quest Book, 1978.
4. Leichtman, R. & Japikse, C. *The Light of Learning - Activating Our Divine Possibilities.* Ariel Press, 2000.
5. Mayer, Elizabeth L., Ph.D. *Extraordinary Knowing - Science, Skepticism, and the Inexplicable Powers of the Human Mind.* Bantam Books, 2007.
6. Orloff, Judith, M.D. *Intuitive Healing - 5 Steps to Physical, Emotional, and Sexual Wellness.* Times Books, 2000.
7. Sugrue, Thomas. *There is a River - The Story of Edgar Cayce.* Holt, Rinehart & Winston, 1942.

Chapter 16. Dreams reveal causes and cures. Page 148

1. Bailey, Alice A. *Esoteric Psychology II.* Lucis Publishing Co., 1936.
2. Corrier, Dr. Richard & Hart, Dr. Joseph. *The Dream Makers.* Bantam Books,
3. Faraday, Ann. *The Dream Game.* Harper.
4. Hall, Manly P. An Introduction to Dream Interpretation. Pacific Publishing Studio.
5. Sechrist, Elsie. *Dreams - Your Magic Mirror.* O. Cowles Books.
6. Thurston, Mark A., Ph.D. *How to Interpret Your Dreams.* A.R.E. Press.

Chapter 17. The role of healers in self healing. Page 154

1. Hopking, Alan. *Esoteric Healing - A Practical Guide Based on the Teachings of the Thibetan in the Works of Alice A. Bailey.* Blue Dolphin Publishing, 2005.

2. Kirkpatrick Sidney. *Edgar Cayce: An American Prophet.* The Berkley Publishing Group, 2000.
3. Kirkpatrick, Sidney. *True Tales from the Edgar Cayce Archives*, A.R.E. Press, 2015.
4. Leichtman, Robert, M.D. *The Psychic Life - Seeing Beyond the Mundane.* Enthea Press, 2006.
5. Mayer, Elizabeth L. Ph.D. *Extraordinary Knowing - Science, Skepticism, and the Inexplicable Powers of the Human Mind.* Bantam Books, 2007.
6. Meek George W. *Healers and the Healing Process.* The Theosophical Publishing House, 1977.
7. Orloff, Judith, M.D. *Intuitive Healing - 5 Steps to Physical, Emotional, and Sexual Wellness.* Times Books, 2000.
8. Smith, Malcolm. *Spiritual Power Healing Hands.* A.R.E. Press, 2009.
9. Worrall, Ambrose and Olga. *The Gift of Healing - A Personal Story of Spiritual Therapy.* Ariel Press, 1965.

Chapter 18. How to assemble a team of professional practitioners. Page 161

1. Canfield, Jack. *The Success Principles - How to Get From Where You Are to Where You Want to Be.* Harper Collins, 2005.
2. Helms, Joe, M.D. *Getting to Know You: A Physician Explains How Acupuncture Helps You Be the Best You.* Medical Acupuncture Publishers, 2007.
3. Riordan, Hugh D., M.D. *Medical Mavericks.* Bio-Communications Press, 2005.
4. Siegel, Bernie, M.D. *How to Live Between Office Visits.* Harper Collins, 1993.
5. Weeks, Nora. *The Medical Discoveries of Edward Bach, Physician.* Keats Publishing, 1973.

MOBIILIZE THE WILL TO HEAL
Chapter 19. How to pray for healing and wholeness. Page 171

1. Bennett, William J. *The Book of Virtues.* Simon & Schuster, 1993.
2. Cayce, Edgar *Soul & Spirit - Fully Understand Yourself and Your Life.* A.R.E. Press, 2006.
3. Dossey, Larry, M.D. *Prayer is Good Medicine - How to Reap the Healing Benefits of Prayer.* Harper Collins, 1996.
4. Halberstam, Yitta & Leventhal, Judith. *Small Miracles - Extraordinary Coincidences From Everyday Life.* Halberstam & Leventhal, 1997.
5. Ironson, G. & Schneiderman, N. *Cognitive-Behavioral Stress Management (Treatments That Work).* Oxford University Press, 2007.
6. Leadbeater, C.W. *Invisible Helpers.* Theosophical Press, 1896.
7. Leichtman, Robert, M.D. *Fear No Evil - Using the 23rd Psalm for Healing and Self-Renewal.* Ariel Press, 1998.
8. Leichtman, R. & Japikse, C. *Making Prayer Work.* Ariel Press, 1988.
9. Miller, Robert N. Ph.D. *Miracles in the Making - Scientific Evidence for the Effectiveness of Prayer.* Ariel Press, 1996.
10. Underhill, Evelyn. *The Spiritual Life.* Ariel Press, 2000.

Chapter 20. How to link the heart and mind to the soul. Page 178

1. Bailey, Alice A. Discipleship in the New Age. Lucis Publishing, 1944.
2. Blavatsky, H.P. *The Voice of the Silence.* Theosophical Publishing House, 1889.
3. Clemmons, Thomas E. *Relaxation and Meditation.* Waldemar Argow, 1976.
4. Gibran, Kahlil. The Earth Gods. Knopf Press, 1931.
5. Japikse, Carl. The Story of God - What to Say When Asked: "Who is God?" Enthea Press, 2004.
6. Japikse, Carl. *The Light Within Us - A Step-By-Step Guide to Spiritual Growth.* Ariel Press, 1987.

7. Koenig, Harold G., M.D. *Spirituality in Patient Care - Why, How, When, and What.* Templeton Press, 2002.
8. Leichtman, R. and Japikse, C. *Active Meditation - The Western Tradition.* Ariel Press, 1982.
9. MacDonald-Bayne, Murdo. *Divine Healing of Mind and Body.* Ariel Press, 2012.
10. Wilhelm, Richard. *The Secret of the Golden Flower - A Chinese Book of Life.* Harcourt, Brace & World, 1931.
11. Willing, C.A. *The Impersonal Life.* Sun Publishing, 1941.
12. Wing, R.L. *The I Ching Workbook.* Doubleday & Company, 1979.

Chapter 21. The healing effects of movies, music and art. Page 185

1. Atukagawa, Ryunosuke and Kuwata, M. *Rashomon and Other Stories.* Liveright Publishing, 1952.
2. Botton, Alain de, Armstrong, John. *Art as Therapy.* Phaidon Press Limited, 2013.
3. Campbell, Don. Music Physician for Times to Come. Quest Books, 1991.
4. Campbell, Joseph. *Hero of a Thousand Faces.* New World Library, 2008.
5. Heline, Corinne. *Color and Music in the New Age.* New Age Press, 1964.
6. Howard, Ron. Director of Cocoon.
7. Jung, C.G. *The Spirit in Man, Art, and Literature.* Princeton/Bollingen, 1966.
8. Progoff, Ira. *The Intensive Journal Workshop.* Tarcher/Putnam, 1975.
9. Spann, Chip & Haag, Jan. *Blood on the Page.* LAMP, 2006.

Chapter 22. Finding nature's healing energies. Page 197

1. Bach, Edward and Wheeler, F.J. *The Bach Flower Remedies.* McGraw-Hill, 1997.

2. Boone, J. Alan. *Kinship With All Life*. Harper & Row, 1954.
3. Cummings, Stephen and Ullmann, Dana. *Everybody's Guide to Homeopathic Medicine*. Tarcher/Penguine, 1997.
4. Leadbeater, C.H. *The Hidden Side of Things*. Theosophical Publishing, 1902.
5. Leichtman, R. & Japikse, C. Companions in the Light - Interacting with Other Kingdoms of Life. Ariel Press, 2009.
6. Maslow, A.H. *Religions, Values and Peak Experiences*. Atlantic Books, 1994.
7. Tompkins, Peter. *The Secret Life Plants*. Harper and Row, 1972.

Chapter 23. The end of life is a new beginning. Page 205

1. Alexander, Eben, M.D. *Proof of Heaven - A Neurosurgeon's Journey into the Afterlife*. Simon and Schuster, 2012.
2. Amatuzio, Janis, M.D. *Beyond Knowing - Mysteries and Messages of Death and Life from a Forensic Pathologist*. New World Library, 2006.
3. Canfield, Jack, Hansen, Mark & Newmark, Amy. *Miraculous Messages from Heaven - 101 Stories of Eternal Love, Powerful Connections, and Divine Signs from Beyond*. The Donohue Group, 2013.
4. Edward, John. *After Life - Answers From the Other Side*. Princess Books, 2003.
5. Feather, Dr. Sally Rhine, Schmicker, Michael. *The Gift - ESP, the Extraordinary Experiences of Ordinary People*. St. Martin's Press, 2005.
6. Leichtman, R. M.D. and Japikse, Carl. *The Role Death Plays in Life*. Enthea Press, 1987.
7. Leichtman, R. M.D. *Recovering From Death and Other Diseases - Activating Your Daedalus actor*. Ariel Press, 2000.
8. Moody, Raymond. *Glimpses of Eternity - An Investigation into Shared Death Experiences*. Random House Group, 2010.
9. Moorjani, Anita. *Dying to be Me - Journey From Cancer, to Near Death, to True Healing*. Hay House, 2012.

10. Neal, Mary C., M.D. *To Heaven and Back - A Doctor's Extraordinary Account of Her Death, Heaven, Angels, and Life Again.* WaterBrook Press, 2001.
11. Van Praagh, James. *Heaven and Earth - Making the Psychic Connection.* Simon and Schuster, 2001.

This book is a step by step guide that identifies sources of healing and how to mobilize them. It addresses the whole person body, heart, mind and spirit. It draws upon the experiences of thousands of patients, scientific studies, professional observations and personal experiences. The uniqueness of this book is that it encompasses a holistic view to healing and wholeness. Within each of us are layers of function from the concrete physical to gradually increasing subtle levels of feeling, thought, beauty, love, wisdom and joy. As we commune with, integrate and apply these energies, healing transformation can occur.

For physical health there are guidelines on nutrition, exercise, the use of supplements, hormones, and sleep. For emotional health there are compelling discussions of stress, relaxation, and resistance to healing. For increasing mental agility there are comprehensive suggestions for healing memories, incubating healing dreams and enhancing intuition. The spiritual aspects of healing are addressed with enlightened perspectives on communing with nature, prayer, meditation, death and the afterlife.

James L. Kwako, M.D. is a family physician who has been practicing medicine for over 45 years. He has been medical director of the Shealy Pain and Stress Center and Meadowlark Retreat Center. He has been an Instructor at Santa Barbara City College for many years, now called the Center for Lifelong Learning. He has been a Board Member of the American Holistic Medical Association, the Santa Barbara Chapter of the International Association of Near Death Studies and Unity of Santa Barbara. He is founder of the Holistic/Integrative Medicine Study Group of Santa Barbara. He is very grateful to be the father of two wonderful sons and a loving, supportive wife. His email is jameskwakomd@yahoo.com.